EMBODIED BOOKS

Medical Humanities: Criticism and Creativity

Vol 3

Series Editors: Maria Vaccarella, MA, PhD, Senior Lecturer in Medical Humanities, University of Bristol and Kimberly R. Myers, MA, PhD, Professor of Humanities and Medicine, Penn State College of Medicine

PETER LANG
Oxford - Berlin - Bruxelles - Chennai - Lausanne - New York

EMBODIED BOOKS

EXPERIENCING THE HEALTH HUMANITIES THROUGH ARTISTS' BOOKS

Darian Goldin Stahl

PETER LANG
Oxford - Berlin - Bruxelles - Chennai - Lausanne - New York

Bibliographic information published by the Deutsche Nationalbibliothek.
The German National Library lists this publication in the German National Bibliography; detailed bibliographic data is available on the Internet at http:// dnb.d- nb.de.

A catalogue record for this book is available from the British Library.

Library of Congress Cataloging-in-Publication Data

Names: Stahl, Darian Goldin, 1989- author.
Title: Embodied books : experiencing the health humanities through artists' books / Darian Goldin Stahl.
Other titles: Book as body
Description: Oxford ; New York : Peter Lang, [2024] | Series: Medical humanities : criticism and creativity, 2504-5229 ; vol no. 3 | Revision of the author's thesis (doctoral)—Concordia University, 2021, under the title: Book as body : the meaning-making of artists' books in the health humanities. | Includes bibliographical references and index.
Identifiers: LCCN 2023054893 (print) | LCCN 2023054894 (ebook) | ISBN 9781800798168 (hardback) | ISBN 9781800798175 (ebook) | ISBN 9781800798182 (epub)
Subjects: LCSH: Artists' books—Psychological aspects. | Communication in art. | Medicine and art. | Arts medicine. | Communication in medicine. | Sick in art. | Diseases in art.
Classification: LCC N7433.3 .S73 2024 (print) | LCC N7433.3 (ebook) | DDC 495.15—dc23/eng/20240202
LC record available at https://lccn.loc.gov/2023054893
LC ebook record available at https://lccn.loc.gov/2023054894

Cover image: Darian Goldin Stahl, "Field Notes: How to Be With," Artist's Book, Encaustic transfer, monoprint, and silkscreen on silk and handmade paper, 8" round, 2020. Image courtesy of the artist.
Cover design by Peter Lang Group AG

ISSN 2504-5229
ISBN 978-1-80079-816-8 (print)
ISBN 978-1-80079-817-5 (ePDF)
ISBN 978-1-80079-818-2 (ePub)
DOI 10.3726/b19581

Published by Peter Lang Ltd, Oxford, United Kingdom
info@peterlang.com - www.peterlang.com

This publication has been peer reviewed.

This book is dedicated to my sister, Devan Stahl,
and to all those who choose to put their bodies into books.

Contents

Figures

Acknowledgments

There are many people who provided their guidance in the pursuit of this unusual intersection of handmade books and health research. I must thank my PhD supervisory team who gave their enduring support for over five years and ultimately shaped the outcomes of this research-creation project. First, Dr. Kim Sawchuk, who deftly mentored the development of my methodology, invited me to raid her library, and always pushed me to think through the process of making. To Dr. Kathleen Vaughan and Ingrid Bachmann for challenging my pedagogical methods, technical skills, and writing. Lastly, to Dr. David Howes for supporting the vital international fieldwork that comprised much of this book. I must also acknowledge the support of Peter Lang International Academic Publishers editor Dr. Laurel Plapp, the peer reviewers, and the *Medical Humanities: Criticism & Creativity* series editors Kimberly R. Myers and Maria Vaccarella, who fine-tuned the direction and scope of *Embodied Books*. I am eternally grateful for the brilliant critiques and reflections on my work from each of these scholars.

Embodied Books is comprised of numerous collaborators who generously lent their voices and expertise to this research. Scientists Karen Carvalho, Dr. Sofia Granados, and Dr. Hugh Clark trusted an artist to reside within the McGill University Fertility Research Laboratory, and invited me to witness the creativity and motivation present in this space. The scholars I interviewed provided generative perspectives into the concept of art and health that would not have been possible otherwise: Joanna Baines, Christine Borland, Veronique Chance, Egidija Ciricaite, Paul Crawford, Melanie Grant, Fiona Johnstone, Claire Jones, Chisomo Kalinga, Jane Macnaughton, Ariane Mildenburg, Cathleen Miller, Eleanor Perry, Katherine Rawling, Rutherford, Curie Scott, Charlotte Sleigh, and Maria Vaccarella. Dr. Stella Bolaki supervised and partnered with me to conduct the UK fieldwork that shaped this research, and with whom I share a passion for artists' books. Her efforts to assemble the Prescriptions Collection of artists' books set the stage for this investigation.

For the imagery within *Embodied Books*, I am especially grateful for the artists who allowed me to reproduce images of their books, including Veronique Chance, Amanda Couch, Tangy Duff, Jenny Lin, Joan Lyons, Mary Rouncefield, Erin K. Schmidt, and Alan Hall, who represents the eternal artwork of his late wife, Martha Hall. Further, the "Book as Body" workshop participants generously bought into the idea that they could express their symptoms within artists' books. It was the analysis from these group critiques that generated the most vital evidence for *Embodied Books*. Most of all, I acknowledge the long-standing collaboration with my sister, Dr. Devan Stahl, who invites me to use her medical scans within artwork. The generosity of sharing her stories and medicalized body not only motivates this research but also continues to build community with all those who have lived experiences of illness.

I also extend my sincere gratitude to SSHRC Vanier, Mitacs, Hexagram, Milieux, the Carolyn and Richard Renaud endowment, the Rose and Leon Zitner endowment, and the Concordia University Humanities PhD program for funding and supporting wonderfully unconventional interdisciplinary research-creation like mine. These programs prove there is space for the thinking that occurs during artful making and play within academic scholarship.

Finally, I give my deepest gratitude to my friends and family who never questioned my pursuit of the arts, even when they have taken my far away from home. And to my husband Julien Pestiaux, who did not baulk, even for a second, as I turned our entire small apartment into a make-shift art studio so I could complete my artist's book, *Field Notes: How to Be With*, during the Covid-19 shutdowns. I am eternally grateful for your unending enthusiasm and love that buoys my dreams.

Introduction: *Embodied Books*

A book is a body. Even the very language used to describe books reveals our bodily relations with them. Books contain a head, headers, and headbands; footers, joints, a spine, face, and back. The materials bookmakers employ have parallel corporeal significance: signatures, guillotines, scalpels, and bone folders. Books are enveloped in leather or cloth, then placed within jackets to keep them protected. Engaging with a book is then an activation of bodies. Far from an inert activity, reading a book is an embodied performance of cracking its spine, skimming pages, skipping over sections, flipping through chapters, or diving into a good read. Our bodies leave an impression on the books that we hold dear. Our oily fingerprints yellow the corners of pages, creating a pallor and texture like an aging complexion; and the well-worn creases we impart to our most beloved books evoke the wrinkles inscribed on the surface of skin.

As shareable objects, books join bodies together through time and space. Books capture a time of the author, require time from the reader, and yet, resist time entirely as an archival medium. They mediate the wide spaces between the writer and reader as they entangle the perception and imaginations of both parties. Books then take on a life of their own. They seem to possess a self-determined quality as they pass from hand to hand or journey to reside in far-reaching collections. From any distance, books intermingle the consciousnesses of the author with every subsequent reader—a connection that is made all the more meaningful and significant if that book was carefully and lovingly crafted by hand.

My first *artist's book*, that is, fine art that takes on the format and concept of a book, was an attempt to understand another person's body better—that of my sister, Devan. Six years after her diagnosis of multiple sclerosis in 2009, Devan procured and shared with me several complete sets of her MRI scans that her neurologist copied onto a CD. Devan thought, since I was a printmaker studying the medium's connection to medical history, that I could somehow use these biomedical images in my work. Eagerly scrolling through the black and white digitization of her body, I was first struck by how alien these scans felt. Grotesque slices of Devan's face revealing her nasal cavities, cutting through her eyes, and exposing her brain tissue ensured I could not recognize my own sister's face. Although abstract portraiture can similarly evoke a sense of alienation, the artist's hand imbues emotion, storytelling, and context to their visual choices while also inviting viewers into an open-ended interpretation to the work's personal significance. These images, on the other hand, have a singular purpose: to alert Devan's neurologist to the lesions along her brain and spine. I felt a sense of injustice that these scans could only confirm a diagnosis while communicating absolutely nothing about the life-altering consequences of her prognosis, the impact on Devan's sense of identity, nor what it felt like to live daily with the symptoms of MS. I longed for these medical portraits to communicate more.

I was then struck by the seeming pagination of Devan's body within this digital format. As I scrolled my cursor up or down, layers of her anatomy were stacked or peeled away. I imagined that every minute slice of her MRI scans was a piece of paper that could be compiled, bound, and then pulled across my thumb to form the animated illusion of a flip book. With that thought, I felt compelled to materialize these digital scans into an artist's book (see Figure 0.1). Devan's illness narrative could then be printed alongside the images of the body to rectify the absence of identity and voice in her original MRI scans. We could then share these artist's books with others as a dispersed edition in the hopes of giving support to others who have felt similarly diminished by medical scans, as well as educating physicians on the impact medical scans can have on the patient's sense of self.

Our collaboration bloomed into a rich, reciprocal practice of making and reflection. We began to interweave our respective interdisciplinary backgrounds in medical ethics, religion, printmaking, art education, and communication studies into the meaning of these creations, and how each of these disciplines affords us lenses through which to view the artist's books. It is also a collaboration that enables us to speak more directly to each other about difficult topics like illness when there is an artist's book between us. Ultimately, I understand the labor required to transform Devan's body into

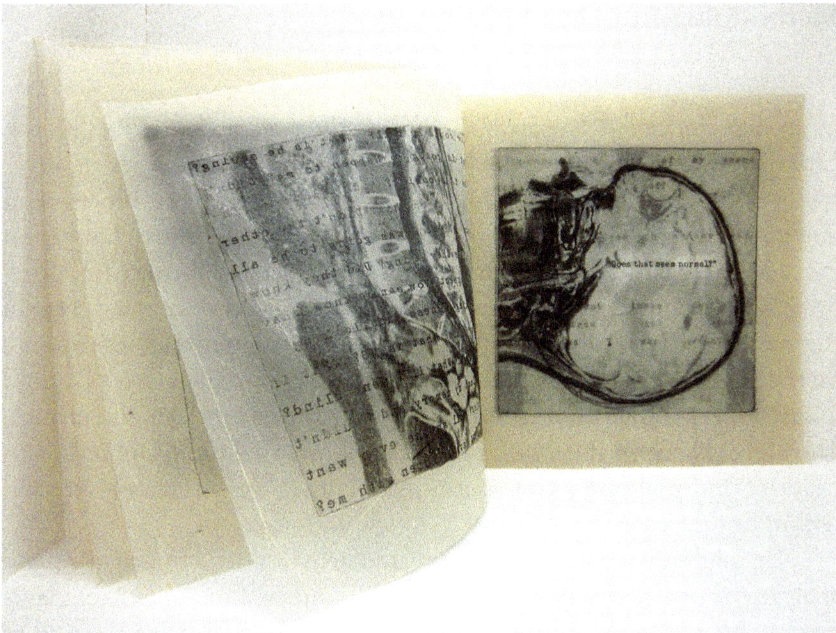

Figure 0.1: Darian Goldin Stahl, *The Importance of Dualism*, Photo-intaglio on waxed silk tissue Gampi paper, 6″ × 5.5″, 2014.

a book to be a gesture of my care: to let her know I am deeply considering the impacts of a diagnosis on her life and, in a small way, bending the world she moves through toward more empathetic understandings of what it is like to live with illness—one artist's book at a time.

Embodied Books emerges from this initial collaborative bookmaking practice and expands to include how others employ artists' books to express their lived experiences, communicate with their physicians, critique harmful Western medical paradigms, and point toward a more collaborative and creative future in health research and education. I use a combination of artistic, philosophical, and field research to investigate the potential of this medium as a primary resource in health and illness research. The core argument of this monograph is that artists' books are uniquely suited to educate readers about bodies by engaging their sensing bodies.

Methodology and Methods

In my experience as a fine art health humanities researcher and educator, I have found a dearth of research and pedagogies that mobilize *research-creation*, that is, the methodology of learning through the process and outcomes of creating art, within healthcare contexts. Research-creation takes up the call of other health humanities scholars to form critical, theoretically grounded approaches to the intersections of art and health. Rather than simply promoting the sense of wellbeing that arises through exercising creativity, I am investigating if and how critical artists' books might foster critique, dialogue, and learning to enact meaningful change. Therefore, I aim for this book to provide substantial philosophical justifications and pragmatic considerations for integrating research-creation within health research.

Throughout my fieldwork, I created artist's books to organize and analyze the qualitative data I collected. I found creating books that layer textual, image-based, and sensory research to be an effective method of entangling interdisciplinary concepts. Centering bookmaking research-creation throughout my investigation led to new insights into how, for example, scent can enact caretaking for readers, or how nonhuman beings become implicated in the study of human bodies. Once research takes on the form of a tangible object, the initial proposition that an embodied engagement with artwork fosters meaning-making that could not be ascertained through more traditional means of knowledge dissemination alone (like this written book) becomes demonstrably evident. Ultimately, reading and making artists' books became the primary evidence for the effectiveness of research-creation in the critical health humanities.

The initial question driving this research is, "How can artists' books effectively communicate the wide range of lived illness experiences?" Illness is a vast topic and universal condition, yet effects each person uniquely. Given the variabilities of illness, I argue that the multimodal openness of artists' books, such as the intermingling of text with collage, photography, painting, drawing, printmaking, sewing, materiality, and more, is suited to accommodate the variability of sensory methods a person may require to express themselves with fidelity, meaning, and impact. I am also interested to discover if the *process* of translating one's ill body into an artist's book informs or even transforms one's sense of identity and agency.

From a relational standpoint, does reading and experiencing artists' books foster empathy with those who live with illness? If so, how can philosophy help us to contextualize meaning-making and the sense of connectedness while engaging with artists' books? This book, as well as the research-creation produced alongside it, examines if relationality can be fostered with those who experience illness through the embodied processes of making and sharing artists' books.

My goal is not only to investigate what artists' books can offer makers but also how these artworks may go on to impact and sensitize health practitioners. To this end, I examine how teaching bookmaking within a health humanities context can promote criticality and empathy with those who live with illness. Artists' books are a means to create empathy between patients and healthcare professionals (as well as the general public) when they actively address the disconnection between medical diagnoses and the embodied, lived experiences of illness. As medicine becomes more and more technologically mediated, a return to embodied forms of learning through touch, temporality, and gesture within the intimate sensory engagement of artists' books helps to mend the epistemic gap between treating and living with illness.

The methodology I use to situate the allure and power of artists' books to form embodied connections between makers and readers is phenomenology. A phenomenological practice is apt for this investigation because it examines lived experiences, and in particular, re-examines habituated phenomena. This reexamination is especially significant when the matter at hand concerns how the body changes in times of illness. Likewise, phenomenology is useful to examine how artists alter the typical reading and format of books to indicate the ill body. Contemporary critical[1] and

1 Lisa Guenther, "Critical Phenomenology," in *50 Concepts for a Critical Phenomenology*, eds. Gail Weiss, Ann L. Murphy, and Gayle Salamon (Evanston: Northwestern University Press, 2020), 11–16.

feminist[2] phenomenology provide further frameworks for reexamining lived experiences that are cognizant of how identity subjectively influences perception in order to promote productive change and more inclusive practices within fields like healthcare.[3] Explicit acceptance of subjectivity in the topics of health and illness is crucial to our discussion of artists' books because, as the ill body is translated and abstracted into the structure of a book, it is then up to every subsequent reader to interpret meaning from these hermeneutical objects. The ability to evoke a multiplicity of personalized significances forms the basis of the connective power of artists' books that keeps the medium lively and impactful. Artists' books that take on the form of the (ill) body, as well as books that are literally composed of body parts, will be examined as evidence for generative research-creation and phenomenological practices.

Audience and Contributions to Knowledge

The interdisciplinary nature of *Embodied Books* means that anyone who has experiences or interest in art, bookmaking, illness, and/or healthcare will find value in this work. I envision readers to include ill persons, caretakers, healthcare workers, health researchers, healthcare students, librarians, artists, curators, instructors, and all of the overlaps between these categories. For those interested in creation, I go into detail on how to make and interpret artists' books. I aim for the full range of makers, from those with little-to-no artistic background to extensive artistic practices to be well equipped to create a meaningful artist's book by the end of this

2 Linda Fisher, "The Illness Experience: A Feminist Phenomenological Perspective," in *Feminist Phenomenology and Medicine*, eds. Lisa Folkmarson Käll and Kirstin Zeiler (Albany: SUNY Press, 2014), 33–52.

3 Further reading on the topics of feminist phenomenology include Gail Weiss, *Intertwinings* (Albany: State University Press of New York, 2004); and Elizabeth Grosz, The Volatile Bodies: Toward Corporeal Feminism (Bloomington: Indiana University Press, 1994).

read. Considerations for collection and display of artists' books will prove useful for art and library workers who wish to proliferate the medium for general or targeted audiences. For scholars, I provide philosophy and theory on the relational power of artists' books. Healthcare practitioners may utilize *Embodied Books* to become more attuned to the nonlinguistic, creative ways patients may express themselves. For instructors, I provide a step-by-step case study for conducting bookmaking within medical humanities classrooms. In all of these topics, I detail the pitfalls one may encounter and methods to overcome these challenges so readers will feel empowered to take up this medium and experience it for themselves.

Embodied Books primarily engages the disciplines of artists' books, the phenomenology of illness, and the critical health humanities. As artist's book scholars like Stefan Klima,[4] Charles Alexander,[5] Joan Lyons,[6] and Johanna Drucker[7] point out, the medium has had fluctuating appeal since its conception in the 1970s, which has resulted in a scarcity of literature on the topic from philosophical and sensory perspectives. However, the diversification of the artist's book genre, recent appeal to university library holdings, and uptake by women in particular have led to a resurgence of the medium for the twenty-first century. Most of the publications concerning artists' books focus on the art history and categorization of the medium, but what is far less analyzed is their philosophical precedent for empathy creation. As artists' books become more well known, it is vital to set a methodological foundation on which to contextualize their potential within other fields of research, such as healthcare.

With regard to artists' books on topics of illness, a foremost scholar is Stella Bolaki, who is the principal investigator for the Prescriptions Collection held at the University of Kent.[8] This project collected over

4 Stefan Klima, *Artists Books: A Critical Survey of the Literature* (New York City: Granary Books, 1998).

5 Charles Alexander, *Talking the Boundless Book: Art, Language and the Book Arts* (Minneapolis: Minnesota Center for Book Arts, 1995).

6 Joan Lyons, *Artists' Books: A Critical Anthology and Sourcebook* (New York: Visual Studies Workshop Press, 1985).

7 Johanna Drucker, *The Century of Artists' Books* (New York: Granary Books, 1995).

8 Stella Bolaki, "Artists' Books and Medical Humanities," *Journal of Medical Humanities* 41 (2020).

seventy artists' books on the broad topics of health, illness, and mortality.[9] I conducted fieldwork in this collection, and many of these artists' books are cited in the following chapters as primary resources.

For the discipline of artists' books, research-creation contributes valuable methodologies for their formation and interpretation. Specifically, I outline the aspects of *bookness*, that is, our engrained and preconceived notions of structures and formats for various books, and how artists manipulate these aspects to engrain meaning. The written word in conjunction with images and an activation of the senses enables multimodal strategies for expression that can hardly be matched by any other medium. When the topic of these works concerns illness, disability, and medical encounters, their potentiality for countering bias and stigma by fostering empathy positions artists' books as a medium of vital significance.

The applied research-creation proposed in *Embodied Books* is a wholly original approach to the phenomenology of illness. Although Merleau-Ponty (and many other phenomenologists since) employs a study of paintings like Cezanne's to conceptualize perception and the (in)visible,[10] I take this practice a step further and ask what the multi-sensory aspects of engaging with artists' books may reveal about the body's perceptual abilities. Additionally, phenomenology aids in conceptualizing how *making* art with and for others initiates an empathetic response between authors and makers. Finally, there has never been an explicit connection made between the caretaking aspect of artists' books and the phenomenology of illness. I argue that creating artists' books with and for others, as my collaboration with my sister exemplifies, is a method of showing care and intertwining phenomenological "flesh," which is a novel contribution to this philosophical space.

The third discipline this research-creation engages is the critical health humanities, which is a broad and inclusive field for critical health research that may fall outside of clinical boundaries. Rather than a set of pedagogies for mobilizing the humanities within medical school, generally known as

9 Stella Bolaki and Egidija Ciricaite, *Prescriptions: Artists' Books on Wellbeing and Medicine* (London: Natrix Natrix Press, 2017).

10 Merleau-Ponty, "Eye and Mind," in *The Essential Writings of Merleau-Ponty*, ed. Alden L. Fisher (New York: Brace & World, Inc., 1969), 259.

medical humanities, the *health* humanities widely applies to health research conducted across any number of disciplines, such as the social sciences, literature, and art.[11] The health humanities recognizes that biology and medicine are but links within a network of factors that determine one's health and wellbeing. Once released from a scientific paradigm, humanities- and arts-based methodologies may be better suited to engage with the social determinants of health and illness, especially in community partnerships. If health professionals aim to cultivate more productive, informed, and aligned partnerships with patients, then an interdisciplinary health humanities approach is integral to such aims.

The *critical* in critical health humanities connotes a turn toward activism and change. Beginning with the notion that previous arts interventions have not been risky or consequential enough to produce changes in healthcare paradigms at the roots of patient and practitioner discontents alike, the critical health humanities investigates how art and humanities approaches might address chronic healthcare issues like systemic pressures for time, suppression of emotion, and unproductive hierarchies. One strategy to keep health research dynamic and reflexive is to integrate interdisciplinary arts-based methodologies that take learners and practitioners out of their comfort zones. Emerging critical health scholarship provided by Paul Crawford,[12] Alan Bleakley,[13] Arno Kumagai,[14] and Jane Macnaughton[15] support such practice-based approaches to health research,

11 Paul Crawford, Brian Brown, Charley Baker, Victoria Tischler, and Brian Abrams, *Health Humanities* (Hampshire: Palgrave Macmillan, 2015), 6.

12 Ibid.

13 Alan Bleakley, "Transitions in Health Humanities—Towards a 'Critical' Health Humanities that Embraces Beauty," in *In/Sight 2: Engaging the Health Humanities*, eds. Lianne McTavish and Pamela Brett MacLean (Edmonton: University of Alberta Press), 12.

14 Arno K. Kumagai, Elizabeth K. Jones, and Anne L. Kittendorf, "Creative Art and Medical Student Development: A Qualitative Study," *Medical Education* 51 (2017): 174–183.

15 Jane Macnaughton and Havi Carel, "Breathing and Breathlessness in Clinic and Culture: Using Critical Medical Humanities to Bridge an Epistemic Gap," in *The Edinburgh Companion to the Medical Humanities*, eds. Anne Whitehead and Angela Woods (Edinburgh: Edinburgh University Press, 2016), 296.

like research-creation, rather than solely the intellectual study of philosophy and case studies. A utility perspective of arts-led pedagogies suggests they can improve communication skills and tolerance of ambiguity, which are two leading causes of medical error.[16] In a more intrinsic evaluation, making space for research-creation enables students to access buried emotions and counter time demands that can ultimately lead to burnout, empathy fatigue, and the perception of indifference from their patients.[17] This book thus explores how critical art practices merge with health research to advocate for meaningful change to benefit both patient and practitioner.

The integration of humanities and arts methodologies in healthcare institutions is gaining momentum. Studying art and visiting museums are on the rise within health humanities syllabi; however, *making* art has yet to find a solid purchase in these classrooms. As well, the growth of the health humanities pedagogies has primarily focused on illness narratives and literature, leaving the power of sensory communication, like that possible in artists' books, generally overlooked. Given the gap of conceptual and practical models for sensory and practice-based research-creation in health contexts, I am in the unique position to connect these fields of study and point its direction for future applications.

Book Structure

The first half of this book is devoted to getting a handle on what artists' books are and what they can do. I set the groundwork for how bodily phenomena are translated into book forms, how centuries of printing and bookmaking have set a visual standard for various types of medical printed matter, and finally, how artists flip these conventions on their heads in order to communicate experiences of illness. A conceptual

16 Alan Bleakley, "When I say … The Medical Humanities in Medical Education," *Medical Education* 49 (2015): 960.

17 Kumagai, Jones, and Kittendorf, "Creative Art and Medical Student Development: A Qualitative Study," 174.

framing of bodily representation in and as books is formulated in these initial chapters, which is then employed to examine concrete examples of artists' books. The last half of this book focuses on specific artworks that exemplify the potentiality of artists' books in the health humanities, including the proliferation of diverse perspectives on health within institutional archives, employing artists' books directly in the clinical setting, and health humanities pedagogical case studies. The narrative arc of *Embodied Books* moves from broad ideas about the book as a body, and concludes with specific examples of student-makers and their books.

Chapter 1 provides a philosophical foundation on which to build the meaning-making of artists' books, namely, phenomenology. The examination of lived experience and sensory evocations of artists' books position phenomenology as an apt framework for this investigation. It is also applied to account for the feelings of connectedness between makers and readers. The chapter is structured in a question-and-answer format, which anticipates the most pertinent questions readers may initially have about artists' books and how they are related to illness. The first question is as simple as, "What are artists' books?" and culminates in the much more complex question, "What do artists' books *do*?" This chapter also outlines the aspects of bookness. Capitalizing on or subverting facets of bookness prevails as the guiding source of influence for artists to overtly and tacitly communicate their lived experiences to readers. The practice of phenomenology is sustained throughout this book as the primary methodology for both creating and reading artists' books.

Chapter 2 outlines the development of artists' books as a discrete medium, paying particular attention to distinguish it from other printed matter that intersects with topics of health and illness. I argue that after a tumultuous start to the medium of artists' books in the 1970s and lofty expectations as a "democratic medium," the contemporary expansion of the genre evidences the grassroots vitality and usefulness of printed matter to build community, educate outsiders, and disseminate ideas on what it looks like to live well. This chapter gives special considerations to the different strategies of acquiring and displaying artists' books in learning institutions, and how collecting a diverse array of artists' books is also a method of decolonizing library archives.

Chapter 3 takes on a longitudinal perspective on the implications of books to disseminate ideas of medicalized bodies. I show how anatomical treatises' images and materials are reproduced through the centuries again and again until the standards for their bookness are set. Artists today then appropriate these historical images and practices in order to reimagine and re-present them according to their own contemporary ethics of care. The main argument for this chapter is that appropriation is a method for artists to critique the cultural legacy of Western medicine, which instilled racist and paternalistic biases that reverberate through time and are still experienced by patients today. To counter these harmful biases, this chapter concludes with methods for productively introducing the critiques offered in artists' books within the medical humanities classroom. Although critique is a standard practice in art and science, integrating such reflexive practices into the culture of healthcare can be met with skepticism and resistance, as medical humanities course feedback surveys indicate. I offer methods to contextualize collaborative atmospheres, overcome some hurdles to student buy-in, and the rationale for mobilizing the arts as a method of cultural growth.

Chapter 4 then examines how specific bookmakers manipulate and subvert the aspects of bookness to communicate their encounters with medicine. This chapter is informed by my fieldwork in the UK as a visiting scholar in the University of Kent Medical Humanities Program, interviews with scholars, and time spent with the artists' books within the Prescriptions Collection. These perspectives frame my subsequent conceptualization on the impact creating artists' books has for the artists' senses of well-being. I evidence how artists seize the authority of "the book" as an icon of knowledge in Western culture either because their illness experiences are too complex and difficult to express through words alone, particularly for experiences like death and dying, or they have felt disempowered within medical systems. Enabling total control over the creation and publication process restores a sense of agency to share their unique and uncensored stances on what it is like to navigate contemporary medicine. To merge all of these voices and artistic perspectives, this chapter is structured as a sensory read-through of my research-creation artist's book, *Field Notes: How to Be With*, which layers interview transcripts and artistic collaborations.

Chapter 5 invests in a close examination of one artist, Martha Hall, and her strategic employment of artist's books within clinical interactions. Hall's practice exemplifies the capacity of artists' books to influence practitioners' understanding of illness, as sharing these books led to more effective communication with the oncologists charged in her care. After Hall's death from a reoccurrence of cancer in 2003, her books have since been used as pedagogical source materials in medical humanities classrooms, where they sensitize future health practitioners to differences in communication styles and expectations for quality time they can expect to encounter with their patients. I argue that spending time with Hall's artist's books is not only a powerful experience of confronting illness and mortality but is in itself a practice to counter some of the most systemic concerns facing medical students. Hall's books show how the accounts of one's life can endure as artist's books, as her legacy continues to foster care and empathy with new generations of health learners.

The final chapter outlines the "Book as Body" artist's book workshops I developed and conducted in Canterbury and Paris as case studies for research-creation health humanities pedagogies. These workshops apply a phenomenological process of making and reading artists' books on the topic of symptoms. After detailing the workshop procedure, I use the artists' books created by the participants as well as transcriptions of our group critiques as evidence that the phenomenological process of creation and reinterpretation offered participants insights into their own experiences and expanded understandings on the impact of symptoms for others. Sharing their books with the other participants ultimately formed a sense of reciprocal caretaking as they spent time engaging with the medical experiences of one another, holding their book-bodies, and engaging in collective meaning-making. This chapter is meant to serve as a replicable model for practice-based approaches to phenomenology and research-creation.

Artists' books are first and foremost an experiential medium whose full meaning can only be grasped by handling them in person. Although there are essential compromises to providing an account of artists' books rather than a direct experience of them, I have sought out permission from each artist to reprint images of their artwork within this book and provide a rich sensory description of each work to make up for these deficiencies. I aim for readers to be inspired to seek out such works in nearby collections in order to experience artists' books firsthand. As well, by providing detailed instructions for making an artist's book on a phenomenon felt within one's body, I aim for readers to try this reflective practice out for themselves. In and through the creation process, we may understand ourselves anew and enable others to understand us for the first time.

CHAPTER 1

How to Read Artists' Books

Introduction

Reading an artist's book on illness is a practice of being with its maker. The artist identifies a bodily phenomenon, imagines its form, labors it into being, and shares this materialization of her consciousness with each reader in an intimate, one-on-one encounter with her book. As an abstract and subjective work of art, the reader is invited to use their sensing body to interpret the artist's book. The aesthetic and sensory choices of the bookmaker initiate the reading, while its significance emerges from the entanglement of each reader's unique background, worldview, and perception of the book-body—leading to a multiplicity of co-created meanings. Artists' books are thus inherently relational, and the bond between bodies that occurs while one holds, senses, reads, and performs another's handmade book is a connective force between two people that is forged again and again, through time, and over any distance.

To conceptualize the power of artists' books to express lived experiences of illness to and with others, I begin this book with an investigation of what exactly artists' books *are* before examining what they can *do*. In the creation process from inception to dissemination, I will employ the most useful terms and practices from related philosophies, namely phenomenology, to make sense of the meaning-making and relational qualities of artists' books.

I situate my study of artists' books on the ill body within the Anglophone Western context, and particularly in regard to collections within the UK, US, and Canada. I include artists' books on the broadest topics of health and illness, including themes of profound or life-long chronic illness, acute or short-term illness, injury, disability, mental illness, bodily distress, dying, mourning, pregnancy, changes to body schema, and medical experiences more generally like doctor–patient encounters. What becomes apparent within these topics is that the books relay not only the effects of illness on the body but also the far-reaching impact of those changes on personal relationships and daily life. I choose this broad scope because of the relatively small number of primary artist's book resources and collections that engage with topics of illness and to promote a wider application of this research. For ease of reading, I include all of these articulations under the title of "illness" with full concessions to the understatement or reductionism of this term.

Additionally, I fully acknowledge that some communities might find this overarching characterization problematic, particularly disability and pregnancy communities who do not identify as ill. Although the histories and contexts of these communities are distinct, changes to bodies often share socioeconomic, political, and relational impacts to lived experiences, and increase the frequency of interactions with healthcare systems. Another overarching link between these topics is a fundamental misunderstanding between outsiders and those directly impacted. For example, although one might be experiencing a disability, there also remains the likelihood for wellbeing and even health—states that may surprise nondisabled people. This is the lens through which I investigate artists' books within the vast topics of medicine. However, I envision a future where each of these categories has its own robust artist's book collection database to employ for equally in-depth investigations.

To structure this initial chapter, I have chosen a "question and answer" format because of the relative newness and obscurity of artists' books as a distinct art form. For instance, although nearly anyone can conjure up numerous examples of famous paintings or sculptures, asking one to name an example of an artist's book is a much harder prompt. I have therefore attempted to anticipate the readers' initial queries of artists' books and thoroughly answer each in order to build a common foundation of discourse for the subsequent chapters.

What Is an Artist's Book?

In the immediate decades after curator Diane Perry Vanderlip coined the term "artist book" in 1973 as a distinguishable medium, much of its mainstream potential has been stymied by critics, curators, artists, and scholars trying to pin down what exactly an artist's book *is*.[1] Even the name for this medium, from book arts, artistic books, and book works, to the controversial inclusion of a possessive apostrophe in artists' books, has been the topic of much debate. In an effort to move well away from this mire and instead focus on the medium's function, I will only briefly touch on its definitions while admitting to this contentious endeavor.

Given the unstable definition of artists' books, it could be simpler to categorize the medium by stating what it is not: a bound collection of photographs or reproductions of an artist's work (also known as a photobook, portfolio, or catalog); a self-published or small press periodical or magazine (known as a "zine"); a handcrafted cover and binding of blank pages (handmade journals or sketchbooks); a handcrafted book containing original prints or illustration alongside another author's text (a handcrafted special edition, edition de luxe, or livre d'artist); text aesthetically arranged on a page (concrete poetry or calligram); or an industrially printed illustrated narrative (also known as comic books or graphic novels). However, even these distinctions are blurry as one could find noteworthy exceptions to each that identify as artists' books. Therefore, I assert that an artist's book, in its broadest definition, is *an object of fine art that conceptually and formally engages aspects of a bookness, typically conceived of and created by a single person.*[2] *Bookness* here connotes any and all culturally engrained preconceptions for how the various forms of printed book media are structured, look, and function. Attempting to taper artists' books under a more focused definition risks limiting the medium's sheer breadth

1 Stefan Klima, *Artists Books* (New York: Granary Books, 1998), 12.

2 This definition has been devised between a number of sources, including Johanna Drucker, *The Century of Artists' Books* (1995); Joan Lyons, *Artist's Books* (1985), and Stefan Klima, *Artists Books* (1998).

of forms and purpose. To keep artists' books dynamic and versatile for their makers and readers, using the most inclusive definition possible will also prove to be the most productive.

When we imagine a book, it typically takes the form of a shallow rectangular object with a stack of paper bound within front and back covers, which is a format known as a codex. The gestures and expectations for book formats are rules that have been forged over centuries of bookmaking traditions until their conventions become completely intuitive for the reader. Turning pages from right to left, reading text from left to right, up to down, graphic black text on white paper, typography, font, embossment, Braille, bullets, columns, text blocks, image blocks, bitmapping, paragraphs, margins, gutters, headers, footnotes, endnotes, bibliographies, and citations; as well as the conventional layouts of novels, magazines, newspapers, catalogs, journals, notebooks, sketchbooks, pamphlets, scripts, comics, cookbooks, children's books, coloring books, pop-up books, flip books, scrapbooks, chapbooks, photo albums, yearbooks, how-to manuals, textbooks, dictionaries, encyclopedias, guidebooks, travel books, language translation books, coffee table books, pocketbooks, rolodexes, flip charts, calendars, scrolls, hymnals, bibles, and more can all be considered articulations of bookness. As you read this laundry list, images of each example may have flashed across your mind that demonstrate the existence of shared preconceived expectations for bookness.

Artist's bookmakers rely on readers intuiting the rules of bookness in order to break them. The rules of bookness have been set in place through centuries of ever more efficient methods of industrialized printing. However, handcrafting a book enables artists to fully manipulate and subvert each aspect of bookness to evoke or disrupt our memories with print media and propel old or new associations. The above examples of bookness all contain their own history and strategies of communicating information, and artists capitalize on that cultural knowledge in the creation of their artists' books as self-referential conceptualizations of how information gets transferred. Conceptually engaging with bookness means employing the idea of "the book" as an iconic symbol of enduring knowledge. For example, sticking to the conventions of traditional leather-backed bookbinding can lend an artist's book a sense of lasting authority, while printing artists' books on newsprint may give the impression of immediacy and disposability. As we will see throughout this investigation, the material and structural choices of artists' books hold unspoken meaning that can be just as significant as what is printed on their pages.

To fully answer what an artist's book is, I next take up the metaphysical significance of creating artwork about and read through the body. Put simply, an artist's book on illness is an extension of the maker's sensing body. A phenomenological framework is helpful to conceptualize how the creation of an artist's book seems to animate a bound stack of pages into a book-body. Phenomenology is a philosophical practice of examining lived experiences in and through the sensing body, which Maurice Merleau-Ponty describes as the intertwining of "flesh" as "an 'element' of Being."[3] Flesh here is not a boundary of skin between the self and other, but the site for the tangible and intangible give and pull of sensation, perception, and understanding between humans and their surroundings. I posit that flesh in this sense can also describe the interaction of bodies through artists' books. The merging of sensory and textual expression held in the artist's book makes this medium an exceptional site for a phenomenological practice.

The circulation of books from hand to hand also supports the notion that artists' books are inherently phenomenological. As flesh radiates and extends our bodies to the limits of our vision, the range of our voice, and the reach of our hands, flesh is reciprocally gathered back into the body through the senses from the things and beings that surround us. Elizabeth Grosz explains that this elemental flesh "does not just clothe subjects, objects, and their relations with its touch; it doubles back on itself as the invisible underside of the visible."[4] This redoubling of flesh is materialized through bookmaking, wherein the flat space of a sheet is suffused with language and sensory information, layered, folded back into itself along a spine, bound into a mass, and finally covered with a thicker skin. This book-body becomes an externalized artifact of its maker's lived experience,

3 Maurice Merleau-Ponty, *The Visible and the Invisible* (Evanston: Northwestern University Press, 1968), 139.

4 Elizabeth Grosz, "Merleau-Ponty, Bergson, and the Question of Ontology," in *Intertwinings*, ed. Gail Weiss (Albany: State University Press of New York, 2004), 23.

the dissemination of which can now greatly extend her flesh's reach. The invisible redoubling of flesh is performed whenever one's artist's book is opened. Such a phenomenological framework gives language and form to the enduring impressions of an artist's book long after its creation, and even after the lifetime of its maker.

The allegory of "body as book" seeps into our common vernacular for how we understand and relate to other people. Emotions can be "read on the face" or secrets exposed by "reading her like a book." Grosz explicitly calls upon the form of books to elucidate the reversibility of flesh: "The body is a page or material surface, possibly even a book of interfolded leaves, ready to receive, bear, and transmit meanings, messages, or signs, much like a system of writing … some of which have been effaced, others of which have been emphasized, producing a body as a text which is as complicated and indeterminate as any manuscript."[5] While Grosz here proposes that the body can be understood as a book, I argue that the opposite is also true: the book is a body. The textual and temporal aspects of the artist's book speak to the reader, while its materiality is taken in through multiple senses—transforming the book into a bodily proxy for the artist who wishes to tell me something about herself. The artist's imagination and labor to create her book-body can then become a part of my own consciousness when its carnal matter merges with mine. The "book as body" allegory is here fully realized as a phenomenological investigation of the visible and the invisible—of elemental flesh. When we attempt to define what an artist's book is, we can now identify this object as an engagement, expansion, and layering of flesh.

Why Artists' Books?

I see artists' books to be an apt creative form to effectively relay lived experiences of illness for a myriad of reasons. First, the sheer versatility and control makers have over their multimodal artists' books ensures that

5 Elizabeth Grosz, *Volatile Bodies* (Bloomington: Indiana University Press, 1994), 117.

they can express the particularities of their experiences (or leave more space for open interpretation) in the manner they see fit. Although artists' books are abstract fine art objects, meant to evoke the same wonder and emotion as any other artistic medium, the media-specific inclusions of text and image provide the artist with more control over the "reading" of their work and the chance of maintaining the particularities of the author's auto-ethnographic investigations of bodily unease throughout the interpretive process. For my focus on artists' books that form embodied connections with their readers, I am most interested in the kind of limited edition, multi-sensory, handmade artists' books that balance poetic and didactic media. Artists' books' accessibility, materiality, mobility, performativity, and intimacy make this medium uniquely suited to foster productive sensory communication on what may be difficult discussions to begin out loud.

Accessibility

The accessibility of artists' books extends throughout their physical creation. Artists' books are highly flexible forms of art because they can be extremely intricate in design and construction, or as modest as a single folded sheet of paper or bound stack of photocopies. It is a medium that, in its simplest form, can be learned in an afternoon. One can then choose the media they are most comfortable with to populate its contents, such as photography, drawing, printmaking, paper crafting, or collage. This last medium is particularly useful for incorporating other ready-made and deeply meaningful artifacts like biomedical scans, family photographs, physician appointment cards, test results, or journal pages. An artist may even choose to incorporate larger objects alongside their book within a book box. If there is a meaningful image or piece of ephemera, chances are there is a way to represent it within one's artist's book.

There is a comfort and familiarity with books that may make this medium more approachable for beginners than say, learning how to paint or draw. Books are one of the first media we engage with as infants and often have continued direct contact with throughout our lives. When prompted to create their own books, makers will already have an idea of what their creations may look like and an understanding of the purpose of books in everyday life: to contain and transfer knowledge. These factors lower the stakes for their creations or the feeling of not having enough "artistic ability" to create a book. The obscurity of artists' books is also helpful in this regard because a new bookmaker will most likely not hold a canon of renowned artists' books in their mind to compare their own novice creations against. Likewise, a reader might not have a sense of needing preparatory knowledge of "art culture" in order to meaningfully engage with an artist's book. Finally, one does not need to possess an understanding of literature to read an artists' book, which often do not include large amounts of text. As artist's book scholar Ulises Carrion attests, our innate ability to create connections between form, image, and text "appeals to the ability every man possesses for understanding and creating signs and systems of signs."[6] The ubiquity of books as a domestic commodity for all ages resists a perceived artistic exclusivity, and may lower the psychological barriers of entry for intrepid makers.

The fact that artists' books are not entirely well known has allowed them to remain dynamic and approachable. Without overarching institutional standards or convention for what an artist's book should look like, pioneering makers are taking the medium in exciting and imaginative directions. Further, it seems the subculture and grassroots positioning of bookmaking allows the medium to be adapted for each maker community. For books on difficult topics like illness, the versatility and accessibility of this medium are crucial for makers to communicate full spectrums of lived experiences based on how they see fit.

Materiality

Artists' books can be said to communicate within an economy of means thanks to the expressive potential of materials not typically found in

6 Ulises Carrion, "The New Making of Books," in *Artists' Books*, ed. Joan Lyons (Rochester: Visual Studies Workshop, 1985), 42.

commercially printed books. Within a handcrafted page, a multiplicity of communications can occur all at once. From the type of paper, color, texture, shape, folds, number of pages, weight, gestures, smells, and so many other nonlinguistic signs, it could take a novel to describe the constellation of sensations and all of their potential meanings from a single page. This medium, in other words, is a compact force for material expression.

The types of materials and printmaking techniques used to construct a book enfold additional layers of meaning and influence. For example, the artist may incorporate traditional book materials to form connections with the history of printmaking and bookmaking: leather binding, marbled paper, gold trim, thick rag paper, linen thread, oil-based inks, moveable type, foil lettering, woodcuts, or engravings. Artists employ these traditional bookmaking materials, now also enveloped within additional notions of wealth and prestige in contrast to industrially printed paperbacks, to imbue their creations with historicity or foster an air of authority. Given the dearth of first-person patient perspectives in the history of preeminent medical publications, such illustrious artists' books, in an attempt to fill in gaps of knowledge of what is like to live with bodily unease, highlight these neglected voices as worthy of equal appraisal in healthcare knowledge, thanks to the choice of materials.

An artist's choice of materials not only indicates the impact of personal or even societal experiences of illness but also demonstrates a consideration for the more-than-human beings that influence global health and wellbeing. As we take seriously the notion that the objects we create have vibrancy and a power influence, so too does an investigation of artist's book materials further expand the impact of the book to the nonhuman beings that went into it. A close consideration of artists' books that employ common bookmaking materials like goat leather covers, fish skin binders, calf skin vellum, rabbit skin glue, cow bone folders, insect-derived pigment, silk, or beeswax brings further awareness to our networks of relations with nonhuman lives. Given the scientific standards of experimentation using a wide variety of animal models for the benefit of pharmacology and human health, artists creating works on the topics of health and illness should likewise be cognizant of what bodies are put forward in their work to accomplish their artistic aims. Artists should consider all of the beings bound together in her book as extensions of the meaning of this work, or else the reader may perform this interpretation and stack unintended associations onto the artist's narrative. As the emphasis of health and illness research expands from the personal and into systemic environmental and social determinants, sustainable material choices highlight a consideration for the ecologies in which we live and operate. With closer attention to our materials, we as artists can make fully informed and ethical choices about what we choose to include in our books, and perhaps forge a new lineage of gentler material practices.

Mobility

One of the goals of this book is to investigate how artworks mediate communication between those who live with bodily unease and the greater public. A key feature of artists' books, as opposed to nearly all other art forms, is their invitation to touch and disseminate as a mobile medium. Although reading an artist's book is generally a one-to-one experience, the editionable, portable, and disseminatable aspects of artists' books make them particularly useful for artists to reach the hands of a great number of people. Books thus have a mobile life: they are pulled off the shelf, handed to a friend, archived in public collections, and exist in many distant locations simultaneously.

The methods of mobility for artists' books have evolved over time. As I will expand upon further in Chapter 2, artists' books could be disseminated directly to subscribers through the mail in the 1970s in an effort to circumvent what was perceived to be an exclusionary professionalized gallery system. Today, artists' books are more likely to circulate in private collections, convention circuits, and, most notably for this discussion, university libraries and museum rare book collections.[7] New archives are forming to acquire artists' books due to their underrepresented perspectives and aesthetic engagement. The Wellcome Trust, renowned British collection of all things artistically

7 Klima, *Artists Books*, 55.

medical, established its own artist's book collection in 2016 in recognition of the unique communicative capabilities of the medium.[8] The goal for these special collections is to make artists' books accessible for researchers and the greater public as first-person resources on experiences of illness and medicine.

Performativity

When learning about another's body, the chance of communicating effectively and fostering an embodied connection with the artist increases substantially if the reader's body is also activated. Artists' books can be seen as a hybrid of sculpture and participatory performance due to the physical and durational aspects of engagement. This is different than other durational artwork like film or theater, where the viewer's role is more that of a passive spectator. The activation of an artist's book, on the other hand, implicates the reader as an essential co-performer in a loosely directed duet. The reader has near-total control over how to engage with the work: she sets the timing based on her own pacing and level of engagement, an artist's book can often be commenced at any point, skipped around, or even flipped through backward. The mix of image, materials, gesture, and text ensures that, more often than not, an artist's book can be "read" in any order and its meaning will still be conveyed. Therefore, artists' books have a flexible performativity that is not restricted to the linear rendition of most other time-based or narrative media.[9] If the aim of a book is to implicate its reader as a co-creator in its meaning, then inviting the reader to engage her own body in the activation of this art is essential to its work.

Opening the cover of an artist's books along the hinge of a spine is not an incidental mechanism to hold pages, but an initiation into a space where a reader performs the transformation of a two-dimensional plane

8 Melanie Grant, interview by Darian Goldin Stahl, March 27, 2019.

9 Klima, *Artists Books*, 64.

into a form with depth and timing. The constant oscillation between flatness and volume exhibits the rhythmic vitality of artists' books, almost like a breath. In the activation of an inert object to an aesthetic work of art that speaks to and with you, the performance of the book-body by the reader's perceiving body makes this communication all the more tangible and meaningful.

Intimacy

Finally, I choose to focus on the medium of artists' books for their potential to foster intimate relationality between makers and readers. This feeling of closeness stems from artists' books ability to form sensory connections between its covers. Holding, reading, touching, smelling, spending time, and moving through a book ensures at least a cursory bodily connection with and through this object. Feeling the folds of paper, it is almost as if your hands might intertwine with those who carefully crafted each page. Feeling the slight breeze of turning pages on your face, enhanced even further if the author imbues the book with a scent, ensures the impact of engaging with the work goes beyond the surface level by entering the interiority of the reader. Sharing breath with an artist's book enables a unique embodiment with these bodily proxies.

The private one-on-one engagement with artists' books also fosters feelings connectedness, like a pleasurable meeting between friends, and furthered by the experience of holding such a rare and valued handmade object. The sentiment of spending one's time and labor to create an object for *you*, some far-away stranger in the future who the author will never meet but nevertheless finds important enough to share the most intimate aspects of her body and lived experiences with, is a humbling gift to receive. The vulnerability expressed in the pages of an artist's book on illness confers a sense of trust that the reader will listen closely, honor the narrative within, and handle this object with care. Along with the use of unique materials and forms that could never be replicated in commercial publishing, the preciousness of this book-body prompts the reader to take great care in their reading.

The intimate charge of an artist's book is furthered by how much the object signifies the body of its author. When one's artist's book conveys the realities of her body, imbued with the consciousness of its author and made material for others to see and feel, it feels natural to view this object as an extension of herself. In this material metaphor, the covers are the flesh that harbor a lifetime of experiences and thoughts, layer by layer, on the pages inside. The enormity of such an invitation to handle this book-body is an intimate, reciprocal act of trust and caretaking.

All this is not to say that artists' books are always effective. One of the greatest strengths of this medium, that it engages a reader through the performance of its reading, can also be a hindrance. Not everyone who looks at art also wants to perform it. The ability to glean meaning quickly or appreciate aesthetics passively in say, a museum setting, is a more common but completely antithetical way of experiencing artists' books. Books request your close attention and above all your time, which can be difficult to secure from busy art-goers when there is so much else to see. Second, in an art market that values grandness and large-scale media to create impact, the very compact nature of bound pages—so useful for storing and transporting this artwork over vast distances—restricts viewing to a small space that may not grab viewers from a distance. Finally, the institutional desire to preserve an artist's book is often at odds with the reader's need to touch and hold it. Glass display cases kill the vitality of performance, spatial and temporal gestures of turning a page, and truncate an intimate engagement of the senses into viewing only a single spread. These reasons are a large part of why the medium has not easily proliferated within museum settings for general audiences. However, finding new venues of dissemination, such as libraries, as well as expanding bookmaking programming in universities and studio workshops, may be more fertile ground for the power of artists' books to proliferate.

What Do Artists' Books *Do*?

Phenomenological Connection

This is the most philosophically important question for our investigation into artists' books. In its most simple answer, artists' books connect people. Artists' books on illness alter how we see and understand altered bodies by intertwining the artist's expression and the reader's interpretation. Artists' books might not actually resemble the things in the world they represent, but they excite our imaginations to connote meaning. Bookmakers transform how illness is represented not only to organize and make sense of their own experiences but also to sensitize and communicate epistemic gaps for others throughout their relational performance.

Once again, I find phenomenology to be an effective philosophical practice to conceptualize the connectivity that occurs while handling another's book. A phenomenological practice prompts one to perceive objects, others, and surroundings through the senses, and to imagine how one is perceived by others. The "reversibility of perception,"[10] that is, the dual property of perceiving and being perceived described by Merleau-Ponty, applies to the maker's artistic choices in anticipation of how her book-body will be perceived by readers. The reader is similarly compelled to ask what kinds of meaning they are meant to glean from the sensory and textual configurations presented to them in the artist's book. In short, I ask, "How do you touch a book, and how does a book touch you?"

In practice, phenomenology is typically a discursive process of feeling, description, and (re)interpretation. But what about the sensations or experiences that are difficult or cannot be put into words? When the topics of discussion concern illness and disability, it is vital to widen our definitions of "communication" to those that are not only read, but imaged, felt, heard, gestured, smelled, or revealed over duration. I thus propose to expand the notion of phenomenology from a *discursive* practice into a *material* one as well. Objectifying experiences in the highly versatile medium of artists'

10 Merleau-Ponty, *The Visible and the Invisible*, 138.

books enables makers to utilize any number of nonlinguistic modalities to best communicate the changes to their bodies with their readers.

Phenomenology, Merleau-Ponty explains, "consists in re-learning to look at the world"[11] that has become routine, habituated, or falls into the background of perception in order to reevaluate and even critique the norms and presuppositions of everyday experiences. Scholars of Merleau-Ponty like Don Idhe and Duane H. Davis explain that initiating a phenomenological practice "involves the transformation of the way we understand our world such that we can be astonished before it—the attempt to see our world as if for the first time, through unjaded eyes."[12] Attempting to behold an object "as if for the first time" is most difficult to do with the things we are most familiar with, like traditional books. Because we have been handling books for nearly all of our lives, so much so that their methods of interaction securely reside within our bodily habitus, the book object itself tends to fall away from active perception when it is simply a vehicle for textual communication. On the other hand, the alternative, variable, and even confounding communication strategies of multimodal artists' books compel a fresh read of these objects as they break our engrained notions of bookness. Therefore, I argue that artists' books spark a phenomenological practice of renewed perception that prompts readers to not only pay closer attention to the text within but also to how the materiality of the book object interacts with and complicates the narrative.

With regard to topics of illness, we can draw connections between how both artists' books and illness alter the habitual gestures and performances of bodies. *Phenomenology of Illness* (2016) author Havi Carel explains that the many changes to one's habitual world in times of illness provide vital philosophical perspectives for examining and scrutinizing the norms that structure our society and to re-examine what it means to live a good

11 Maurice Merleau-Ponty, "What Is Phenomenology?" in *The Essential Writings of Merleau-Ponty*, ed. Alden L. Fisher (New York: Harcourt, Brace & World, 1969), 42.

12 Duane H. Davis, "The Phenomenological Method," in *50 Concepts for a Critical Phenomenology*, eds. Gail Weiss, Ann L. Murphy, and Gayle Salamon (Evanston: Northwestern University Press, 2020), 4.

life.[13] That is, it is easier to notice the everyday when it becomes disrupted. The process of reexamining the givenness of the world can also be experienced in artists' books. As bookmakers subvert our preconceived notions of bookness, they make us keenly aware of how our own bodies have become accustomed to engaging with print media. Disruptions to bookness alter the readers' bodily performance of books, which signal parallel meanings for how the author's bodily habitus has also become disrupted by illness. Therefore, reading artists' books on illness makes us doubly aware of other's lived experiences by both their text and embodied engagement.

To exemplify what artists' books do and how they do it, I will focus on particularly salient and pervasive effects of illness, namely bodily dysfunction and time fluctuations, and their parallel manifestations within artists' books. Phenomenologist and M.D. Drew Leder uses the concept of the "disappearing body" to describe how one does not consciously perceive her body when the will and the body's ability to perform her will are harmonious. Objects can also "disappear" through the skillful incorporation of their mass and function into our bodies' movements.[14] For example, the object-ness of a traditional book tends to fall away as our eyes become accustomed to moving across the page and our hands reflexively turn the pages. It is as if the text floats in space when the book object becomes a part of our habitual, disappearing body.

On the other hand, when the accustomed movements of the body are altered or no longer possible due to impairment, those parts of the body seem to push themselves forward as the objects of full attention. This state of hyper-awareness is what Leder defines as a "dys-appearing body"[15] because the body can be felt to be dysfunctioning in its rebellion against our will. Dys-appearing occurs when the body is in pain, or in social settings when "the body can appear as ill, disabled, aesthetically flawed or socially awkward, objectified or sexualized, or as attracting negative attention from others, as in the experience of shame."[16] Dys-appearance thus encompasses

13 Havi Carel, *The Phenomenology of Illness* (Oxford: Oxford University Press, 2016), 208.
14 Drew Leder, *The Absent Body* (Chicago: The University of Chicago Press, 1990), 17.
15 Ibid., 88.
16 Carel, *The Phenomenology of Illness*, 57.

one's perception of the rebellious body part as well as how one perceives others perceiving that part.

To convey the concept of a dys-appearing body as an artist's book, one might construct a book in such a way as to work against our habituated movements through it. The artist might, for example, change the orientation of her book or the direction of text to disrupt its reading ease. To impart a feeling of frustration, the artist may bind her book in extremely complex, disorienting, or completely unreadable arrangements. An artist may also use unconventional, estranging, or unsettling materials like say, raw meat, to antagonize the reader and compel a bodily reaction. To exemplify this concept, my artist's book, *Crunchy Knees* (2019), imprisons the entire block of pages within a fleshy, waxy fabric to impede any sort of reading (see Figure 1.1). As well, the covers break the convention of flatness as I folded them into a kind of stairway. Holding the book, the reader finds the block of pages crinkle and crunch within their fleshy casing. The sensory elements and performance of this artist's book are meant to convey the qualities of arthritic knees and where the sonic symptoms are typically experienced (going up and down stairs). These communicative strategies deploy atypical navigation and materials, which forces the reader to give her full attention in order to perform it—just as I pay an inordinate amount of attention to my own dys-appearing knees.[17]

In addition to concerns over the body's functionality, S. Kay Toombs also identifies that one's sense of time can radically change as a result of illness.[18] Toombs reports that those who experience intense pain often cannot accurately judge the passage of hourly time. One's sense of time can also be altered on much longer scales. The unpredictability of illness may prevent a person from projecting herself too far into the future, which then compresses her timeline into a sense of "living in the moment." Externalizing these changes of temporality through the material and form of an artist's book, rather than through narrative alone, can foster more embodied accounts of subjective time with those who read them.

17 A more complete sensory description of this work is provided in Chapter 6.

18 S. Kay Toombs, "The Temporality of Illness," *Theoretical Medicine* 11 (1990): 229.

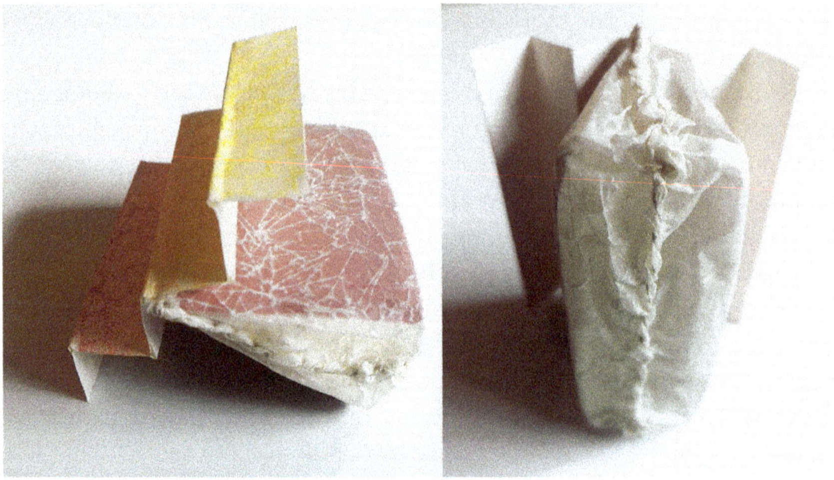

Figure 1.1: Darian Goldin Stahl, *Crunchy Knees*, Waxed silk, paper, plastic sheets, and Caran d'Ache, 6″ × 5″ × 3″, 2019.

The pace and rhythm of reading a typical book are developed for each individual until the repetitive duration of moving one's eyes across and down a page contains a certain amount of predictability. The retention of this bodily habitus is crucial for the artist to then creatively subvert in her manipulation of bookness. For example, the pages may be brimming with dense text and intricate imagery that forces the reader to slow down in order to glean its meaning; or the artist may fill her book with an inordinate number of pages to encourage a durational read. At the other extreme, an artist could make use of a flipbook format to experience her entire book-body in mere seconds. Within my artist's book, *The Importance of Dualism* (2014), I printed the text onto transparent pages (see Figure 0.1). The density of my sister's illness narrative seen through several pages at once gives a sense of attempting to reach into the inscrutable future as well as the frustration of trying to comprehend the present moment. Creatively altering densities of texts likewise alters the viewers' pace of moving through an artist's book, which brings renewed attention to how engrained expectations of temporality also change when experiencing illness.

Thus far, I have focused on the artist's strategies to convey their lived experiences in and through their book works. However, the meaning of artists' books is co-created along with the reader's interpretations. How does the reader's subjectivity influence what artists' books do?

The artistry of this genre occurs in the balance between specificity and openness, which invites the reader to impart her own subjectivity into the meaning of the book. This invitation is what often fosters the sense of connectedness with its maker—as if we are building something together. However, if an artist's book is too didactic, it risks falling into a different category like as a self-published memoir or artfully bound illness narrative, and the reader's role becomes more so that of a passive witness. On the other hand, if it is too abstract, then it ceases to communicate tangible lived experiences of illness to the reader. An artist who seeks to form a relational encounter with her reader must weigh narrative writing and documentary images against poetics, materiality, structure, and the other non-verbal cues for meaning that prompt the reader's interpretation. When one is able to insert their own sense of discovery between the pages of another's book, then this object is capable of mediating a reciprocal dialogue between maker and reader.

The subversion of bookness assists the interpretative potential of reading. The tension between the abstracted book-body the artist presents to us and our own innate expectation for a book to communicate information compels a reader to seek meaning from its strange arrangements. Fracturing normative formulations of bookness shocks the reader into paying closer attention to the significances of the maker's artistic choices. Next, upon reflection, a reader uses the connotations between its form, images, text, and materials derived from her own personal memories and associations to cultivate meaning from an abstract artist's book. Like the practice of phenomenology, artists' books provoke readers to take notice, look upon pages with new sensibilities, and enable our powers of inference to forge our own meaning.

There is no right or wrong way to interpret an artist's book because it is essentially a subjective experience. When a phenomenon is translated and materialized as an artist's book, its reduction to a finite form inversely opens the book to a multiplicity of interpretations. For example, one of my artist's books, *Underlying Traces* (2018), is held within a red velvet-lined box. One might connote sensuality or regality from the inclusion of velvet fabric, but another reader may interpret the use of this fabric as a signal to not touch the book, as it is necessary to protect something extraordinarily fragile. The touch and color of velvet is significant and meaningful, though perhaps differently across any number of readers' own histories, connotations, associations, and backgrounds. When I let my artist's book out into the world, I give up a singular way to read it in favor of forming interconnecting considerations over the ill body. Given phenomenology's assertion that one is the expert of their own lived experiences, it is right to recognize the reader's own understanding of an artist's book as legitimate and true. This hermeneutical openness is key to the connectivity of artists' books. Together, the artist and the reader add layers upon layers of meaning within every artist's book to expand its relational significance.

An artist's book offers one to be in relation with the maker: to read her story, interpret her experience, and care for her book-body. In a close sensory engagement of an artist's book that necessitates interpretation, it is likely that the reader will identify with certain elements that are being portrayed and feel a kinship. However, as Iris Young points out, this feeling of empathy could be ironically rife with misidentification. When readers "imaginatively try to represent to themselves the perspective of members of oppressed groups, too often those representations carry projections and fantasies through which the privileged reinforce a complementary image of themselves."[19] With this pitfall in mind, a better strategy to reading an artist's book is not to necessarily imagine yourself in the artist's position, since it is impossible to fully know another's experience, but instead to come to her book with the expectation of being in productive relation alongside her: to listen closely and be with the themes and sentiments presented.

For all of the productive relationally of fostering phenomenological flesh mentioned thus far, an objection may be that we are not directly engaging with another's body, but through the intermediary of a book. It is fair to ask, "Wouldn't it be better to just tell others directly about your

19 Iris Young, "Comments on Seyla Benhabib, Situating the Self," *New German Critique* 62 (1994): 171.

experience with illness? Why go through the trouble of making a book and risking the reader missing the point?" In response, I have found that if an artist's book sits between a maker and reader as the object of attention, be they close family members like me and my sister or relative strangers, speaking *through* the book, perhaps counterintuitively, allows both parties to speak more directly about sensitive topics than might have been possible otherwise. Artists' books allow one to communicate while circumventing the need for a direct or didactic narrative, which may be difficult or impossible to formulate on particularly emotive topics like illness. Due to stigma, shame, privacy concerns, the desire to keep conversation light and easy, or simply not quite knowing what to say, the empty space between bodies can become a mire. The introduction of an artist's book into this liminality provides a comfortable focus for engagement.

As other scholars have pointed out, particularly post-phenomenologists like Don Idhe[20] and Peter-Paul Verbeek,[21] the self-reflexive focus of phenomenology does not explicitly account for the representation of self through intermediary objects. This is particularly the case for an artist's book, where one builds connectedness *via* her book. The usefulness of post-phenomenology for this discussion of what artists' books do lies in its explicit inclusion of intermediary objects to construct and alter perception. This concept is a productive expansion to our discussion of the phenomenology of artists' books as it turns the focus of inquiry to external objects and media as relational mediations between subjects. If I aim to better understand the lived experience of its maker, then it is essential to actively consider how book-bodies mediate our understanding of another's lived world.

Artists' books are a stepping-stone between silence and openness, from turning away to being with, because illness can be too terrifying a thing to acknowledge directly.[22] An intermediary artist's book breaks the uncomfortable silence around difficult topics, and when most effective, leads to

20 Don Idhe, "Introduction: Postphenomenological Research," *Human Studies* 31 (2008): 1–9.

21 Peter-Paul Verbeek, "Obstetric Ultrasound and the Technological Mediation of Morality: A Postphenomenological Analysis," *Human Studies* 31 (2008): 11–26.

22 Jackie Stacey, *Teratologies* (London: Routledge, 1997), 63.

open and direct communication. It is as if, by sharing an artist's book, the maker is saying, "Although we cannot communicate about this experience directly, either because it is too difficult or because I am not present with you in this moment, read and feel the care I put into this creation so you may know what it is I wish to share with you." Since the ill person has constructed this book herself, the most important things to know about the artist's experience are present at hand.

Fostering Wellbeing

Creative expression is a method of integrating healing for the soul alongside medicine's role of healing the body. What was once hidden or difficult to describe can now be made tangible and experiential as many times as necessary, without the burden of repeatedly retelling what might be a traumatic experience to utter out loud. In a discussion on what artists' books do, it is important to highlight the therapeutic and cathartic effects of creating a work of art that helps both the maker and reader comprehend difficult topics like illness.

The often-random nature of illness can challenge one's most deeply held beliefs and upend what one once thought to be true about her body, relationships, and future. After her own life-altering diagnosis, Carel attests that "such an event challenges the ill person to reflect on her life and search for ways of regaining meaning."[23] Because it is difficult for most people to create meaning from a strictly medical understanding of the body, like the spontaneous proliferation of malignant cells or the development of lesions along the spinal cord, we seek out humanizing metaphors to ground these phenomena within a recognizable paradigm. Artists' books, with their potential for metaphorical expression, re-present the meaning of a diagnosis by rooting it alongside the experience of illness. Creating such organizing objects can foster a sense of order and wellbeing in the midst of unpredictable hardships.

23 Carel, *The Phenomenology of Illness*, 4.

Creating a book is an imaginative and physical labor. Phenomenological bookmaking practices that begin with a series of sensory inquiries prompt one to think deeply about her experience and organize sensations in a way that makes the most sense for her. Even before the process of creation, being prompted to think comprehensively about one's changing body can be a rewarding practice in itself. In her case studies, Carel found that "family, patients, health professionals, carers, and relatives of those who are ill have responded to phenomenological work by saying how positive and useful they found this framework, because it gave clarity and legitimization to their own experiences and thus has lessened their sense of isolation and of being unheard."[24] Practicing a structure for embodied reflection is thus a productive first step to formulating meaning for one's own experiences and communicating illness to others.

Next, the artist must physically labor to create a book-body according to her own point of view. The maker is able to choose how best to compose the experiences of her life across, through, and out of pages, including what complex material metaphors might emerge between its covers. Having full creative agency over how one's body is represented can be a relief. In stark contrast to having very little say over what is revealed in other self-referential media, like biomedical scans, artist's bookmakers *choose* what they deem to be the most important facets of their experiences to portray within their creations. Therefore, one of the vital functions of creating an artist's book on topics of illness is to provide someone who may feel a lack of control over other aspects of her body full and holistic control over the presentation of her body in book form; she may then, if she chooses, invite others to understand her experience as well.

If the maker feels a sense of relief that they are being heard and understood when someone reads her book, then every subsequent reader of the artist's book is actively relieving some distress of the maker. When an artist materializes her experiences into shareable handheld objects, then, as Elaine Scarry conceptualizes, "those objects in turn become the object of perceptions that are taken back into the interior of human consciousness where they now reside as part of the mind or soul, and this revised conception of

24 Ibid., 128.

oneself ... is now actually 'felt' to be located inside the boundaries of one's own skin."[25] The circular movement of unease from internal and invisible feeling, to external and experiential object, and then into a re-internalized perception, transforms pain "from a wholly passive and helpless occurrence into a self-modifying and, when most successful, self-elimination one."[26] As one feels relief by materializing her unease, others can join in further dispersing that sense over a collection of readers who can relate, add meaning, and empathize with the artist through her book.

This is not to say that the sense of care and relief is only one-sided. Engaging with aesthetic media can be a real pleasure, and the materials we choose for our books can be saturated with care for the reader in a very literal sense. Artists may make use of soft materials or perfume their pages to comfort the readers while they navigate the book's difficult terrain. The pages of both *The Importance of Dualism* and *Underlying Traces* mentioned previously are imbued with beeswax and lemongrass oils that waft up to greet the reader and invigorate her body. Or more tacitly, the intention, craft, and labor extended in the creation of an artist's book saturates it with a sense of care for each reader who invests the time engaging with its intricate form. The artist's care is felt even if her physical body is absent, because her creations carry their own message of trust and consideration for whomever the book touches.

Proliferating First-Person Perspectives

Part of what a collection of artists' books on illness *does* is form an archive or catalog of primary, first-person testaments on illness that are authoritative, moving, and impactful for those who have very little knowledge or misinformed ideas on what it is like to be ill. Artists' books have the potential to portray a variety of lived experiences that may counter the readers' expectations of what a body can do and the very definition of a good and fulfilling life.

25 Elaine Scarry, *The Body in Pain* (Oxford: Oxford University Press, 1985), 256.
26 Ibid., 164.

Although illness and disability are universal conditions that will affect nearly everyone if they live long enough, all too often those who do not experience illness or disability formulate their ideas of illness from third-person, inaccurate, or even harmful portrayals in the media. It is therefore likely that a disabled person will experience discrimination and stigmatization, which "can be incredibly costly for the stigmatized person in terms of social relations, but also job prospects, income, and support networks."[27] Objectifying portrayals of atypical bodies constrict the public's conception of illness and disability as simply a series of losses, rather than a valid way of being in the world complete with fulfillment and wellbeing. Put simply, accurate visual representation of illness matters to the perception of illness from general audiences. To counter the misinformation and stigma surrounding illness and disability, self-representing or holistically collaborative artists' books can be a medium to set the record straight on what it is like to live with impairment and, ultimately, cultivate more ethical relationality.

Instead of framing illness as solely dysfunction, Carel makes space for potentially affirmative aspect of illness, whose "positive consequences include improving personal relationships and increased intimacy with family members and friends; a sense of purpose and focus; rediscovering the self; resilience; pride arising from overcoming difficulties."[28] Affirming outcomes from illness and disability are all too often overlooked from those outside of these experiences due to a failure of the imagination to consider the wholeness of a person's life, and not simply this singular aspect. Therefore, when artists' books present illness as a richly aesthetic and sensory object with a full range of ways to interact with the world, then we can also view illness and disability as affirmative ways of being.

Finally, first-person perspectives can also be promoted in collaborative bookmaking practices. If one does not have the dexterity to create a book, then the relational aspect of artists' books is further exemplified in a co-creation process. An artist may seek out a collaboration with family members, friends, physicians, or caretakers to exemplify how illness also engages those around her. Even within fully collaborative practices, however, care

27 Carel, *The Phenomenology of Illness*, 75.

28 Ibid., 126.

must be taken while attempting to portray the lived experience of another person. It is critical to ask:

> What are the politics at play when the primary maker is not part of the community they are representing? Are collaborative partners given parity throughout the process and outcomes of this work? How are subjects compensated and credited? How have the risks of stigmatization or harm in this portrayal been mitigated and accounted for?

Given these potential pitfalls, every standard of ethics must be taken to ensure that members of a collaboration do not end up re-marginalized in the creation of their book. This is not to say that collaborative artworks that portray difference should be avoided, because creating artwork with and for another person can be a worthwhile and fulfilling experience. Ultimately, bearing witness to lived experience and co-creating a book provides the opportunity for all parties involved to practice the caretaking potential of art, to thicken phenomenological flesh between partners, to see and be seen, to touch and be touched by an artist's book.

Conclusion

Western culture's history with print media has set in place a shared understanding for how books look and function, what we deem to be *bookness*; but when artists creatively subvert and alter the facets of bookness to communicate aspects of their lived experiences, then their creations become powerful resources for understanding altered bodies. Phenomenology gives us a useful framework to conceptualize the entanglement of flesh that occurs when holding and reading another artist's book. Artists' books are complex intermediary objects that reach out to be interpreted by others. The aim of conceiving and laboring an artist's book into being is to say something that could not have been possible otherwise, to increase the chance of embodiment by engaging multiple senses, to create an external artifact of lived experience that persists through time and space, and to proliferate ethical relatedness as a disseminated edition. Throughout the remaining chapters, I will continue to hold tension between typical aspects of bookness and how artists manipulate them as I investigate the history of bookmaking and medicine alongside contemporary examples and pedagogical applications of artists' books today.

CHAPTER 2

An Unsettled Medium: The Turbulent Taxonomy and Collection of Printed Matter on Illness

Artists' Books: A Condensed History

While the previous chapter outlined a philosophical understanding of what artists' books are and why they matter, this chapter will help readers recognize and categorize book media as they intersect with topics of illness and medicine. Other authors like Johanna Drucker and Stefan Klima have thoroughly traced the origins of artists' books as a discrete artistic medium,[1] and therefore only a brief summary will be recounted here to contextualize the artists' books I will subsequently unpack. I also seek to distinguish artists' books from their close relatives in this investigation of illness representation, as the book form has proliferated in artistic expression during recent decades. In addition to the genesis of the medium itself, I will also briefly trace the progression of printmaking processes that led to artists' books' production today as these techniques are also intertwined with the dissemination of medical thought.

Because the definition of an artist's book is broad and border crossing, it is impossible to pin down exactly who created the first one. However, one of the first artist's books that resemble our current interpretation of the medium is exemplified by English philosopher, poet, artist, and printmaker William Blake (1757–1827).[2] Although there are an untold number

1 See Johanna Drucker, *The Century of Artists' Books* (1995); and Stefan Klima, *Artists Books* (1998).

2 Betsy Davids and Jim Petrillo, "The Artist as Book Printer: Four Short Courses," in *Artists' Books: A Critical Anthology*, ed. Joan Lyons (Rochester: Visual Studies Workshop Press, 1985), 151.

of extraordinary books aesthetically crafted throughout the centuries prior, Blake's books were unique for their time because they were entirely self-published, the pages were illustrated and editioned using innovative printmaking techniques he invented, and these books were explicitly produced as pieces of art in their totality. Rather than using separated text and image blocks, which became the printing convention with woodcut images and moveable type, Blake organically merged text and image within a single etching plate. Handwritten etched text, à la poupée ink application, and painterly illustrations enabled the visual elements to flow into and inform one another. These techniques stand in stark contrast to the ridged, graphic black lines of letterpress and engraving printing that were much more typical for the time.

In addition to the unique style of printing, Blake's philosophical text is self-referential to the books' printmaking process. For example, in his book, *The Marriage of Heaven and Hell* (1793), Blake makes explicit parallels between etching and the origins of thought:

> But first the notion that man has a body distinct from his soul, is to be expunged; this I shall do by printing in the infernal method, by corrosives, which in Hell are salutary and medicinal, melting apparent surfaces away, and displaying the infinite which was hid. If the doors of perception were cleansed everything would appear to man as it is, infinite.[3]

This passage was in response to John Locke's idea that the soul is a blank slate or white sheet of paper, which would then be written upon through life experiences and the formulation of ideas.[4] In contrast, Blake proposes that a person is more like an etching plate that already contains some incidental and innate impressions, which become more evident and intelligible over time. Blake was thus able to conceive and exemplify his philosophies in and through the bookmaking process—a true indication of an artist's book.

3 William Blake, *The Marriage of Heaven and Hell* (1793), plate 14.
4 Michael Phillips, "'Printing in the Infernal Method': William Blake's Method of 'Illuminated Printing,'" *Interfaces* 39 (2018): 87.

From the invention of moveable type in the Western world around 1450 and until the invention of offset lithography in 1875, bookmaking was a costly and grand affair that consisted of collaborating teams of booksellers, editors, page designers, illustrators, engravers, type setters, printmakers, and book binders, editioned to only a few hundred for their wealthy patrons and subscribers.[5] Book buyers could expect to purchase text blocks from the printer, and take the stack of paper to a binder.[6] Therefore, Blake's one-man operation was quite unique. His self-publishing ventures allowed his philosophies to be printed unedited and without outside commercial pressures. He printed the books as they were ordered, which were admittedly very few, to cut down on his personal production costs. Blake's total control over the bookmaking process is a core feature of the medium that would come to be known as artists' books.

The industrial revolution streamlined book production and drastically decreased its price points. Therefore, any middle-class person could now afford to own books for the first time in history and were encouraged to help themselves to philosophy and literature even without a formal education. As the twentieth century progressed, even more inexpensive forms of printing, like mimeography or xerography, enabled practically anyone to not only build a book collection, but even print editions of simple books for themselves.

The excitement of bookmaking as a new artistic media option took hold in the Russian avant-garde, Futurists, Dada, and Fluxus art movements of the early- and mid-twentieth century. These movements aligned with the anti-capitalist potential of self-publishing low-cost books for the wide distribution of uncensored ideas. Artists employed the handmade book format to subvert the art market's upper-class aesthetic and sensibilities and revolutionize how artwork reached its audience.[7] No longer mediated by curators, these creations could be placed in the hands of audiences directly or even sent through the mail in vast unnumbered editions. The medium

5 Richard Barnett, *The Sick Rose* (London: Thames and Hudson, 2014), 29.

6 Megan Rosenbloom, *Dark Archives: A Librarian's Investigation into the Science and History of Books Bound in Human Skin* (New York: Picador, 2021), 26.

7 Johanna Drucker, *The Century of Artists' Books* (New York City: Granary Books, 1995), 50.

was also taken up by those who had been denied entry into the traditional gallery systems, who then turned to independent publishing as an avenue to reach their audiences.[8] The low barriers of entry for making artists' books, especially with the proliferation of Xerox machines, and the promise of a wide viewership led to this art form being known as a "democratic medium."

However, after their recognition as a new medium and surge of appeal with Diane Perry Vanderlip's curated exhibition, *Artists Books* (sans apostrophe) in Philadelphia in 1973, the popularity and uptake of artists' books floundered.[9] Art critics in the 1970s predicted a space for artists' books alongside airport and drugstore magazine stands, which would enable the general public to easily purchase and own a piece of art.[10] Although self-published artists' editions can today be found in independently owned bookstores and online distributors, the prospect of mass commercial appeal never took root. There are a few reasons for this lack of populist uptake. First, the mimeographed artists' books did not achieve the same shelf-appeal as glossy full-color magazines. As well, the conceptual nature of these publications as a critique of the art market itself did not click with a general audience. To the layperson, these hand-drawn, photocopied, and staple-bound publications appear baffling and somewhat lackluster compared to formally published, hardcover books. Although early proponents of artists' books touted their potentiality as a populist medium, their almost singular appeal to an elite and conceptual art audience proved that this was hardly the case.[11]

A second concern for the medium was the in-betweenness of fine art and book object, which presents challenges for institutions who seek to collect and display artists' books. Galleries and museums work within a mandate to conserve and protect their acquisitions, thereby placing artists' books under glass display cases. Viewers can only stare at a static page of

8 Joan Lyons, "Introduction," in *Artists' Books: A Critical Anthology*, ed. Joan Lyons (Rochester: Visual Studies Workshop Press, 1985), 7.

9 Stephan Klima, *Artists Books: A Critical Survey of the Literature* (New York City: Granary Books, 1998), 12.

10 Lucy R. Lippard, "The Artist's Book Goes Public," in *Artists' Books: A Critical Anthology*, ed. Joan Lyons (Rochester: Visual Studies Workshop Press, 1985), 45.

11 Lippard, "The Artist's Book Goes Public," 48.

these books, truncating the read and prohibiting an embodied experience of them. Alternatively, artists' books may be relegated to the museum library or reading room, which often has different hours, limited access, and does not receive the same kind of public foot traffic as the rest of the museum. At its core, issues of display in museums or galleries present a fundamental contradiction for a medium that was never meant to exist under glass or the halls of museums, but rather to reside in the hands of a reader.

Another reason this medium did not achieve its lofty initial goals is that the economics never added up. Without secure purchase orders from bookstores, artists bore the full upfront expenses of publishing with little chance of selling enough low-price editions to recoup their costs, much less to make a living. Even when the aid of independent artist presses is available, these publication studios come and go as the volatile nature of funding ebbs and flows. As well, it was (and still is) a common practice for artists and galleries to give away simple print publications as a gift for visiting their exhibitions, further undercutting expectations of paying for artists' books. Therefore, it was extremely difficult for artists to form a dedicated, sustainable artists' book practice. Instead, the field was dominated by well-established artists from other media, like Ed Ruscha and his popular artist's book, *TwentySix Gasoline Stations* (1963), who could already afford to produce artists' books to an eager audience. In summary, the notion of mass distribution of low-cost artists' books placed undue economic burdens on the artists to compete with retail publishers for a general audience that simply did not exist.

In the latter part of the twentieth century, the format and definitions for artists' books began to schism and evolve. Expanding from the narrow conception of artists' books as photocopied mass editions,[12] the term also enveloped book objects that embraced sensuous materiality as an additional communication strategy. The proceeding decades saw the rise of more sculptural artists' books that made use of meticulous handcrafted techniques and an attention to the reader's embodied experience—more closely resembling Blake's artist's books than the Fluxus photocopied productions

12 Lucy R. Lippard, *Six Years: The Dematerialization of the Art Object from 1966 to 1972* (New York: Praeger Publishers, 1973), 3.

of the 1970s. Artists' books also became institutionalized within academia. These formal classes and book arts majors tend to be housed within printmaking departments, further cementing the handcrafted and original print associations with the definition of this medium.

To avoid the costly pitfalls of mass production, artists shifted to producing extremely small or even one of kind editions of their books. These types of artists' books, or what Drucker terms *auratic objects*, "suggest a world in which the book is an artifact of winsome, recondite and esoteric, secret and precious, available to the initiate rather than the casual or widespread reader."[13] Prized for their rarity, material aesthetic, and creative experimentation, the auratic artist's book attracts the attention of libraries and private collectors while also commanding significantly higher prices than their forebears, all of which has enabled a new generation of artists to form more sustainable and inventive artist's book practices.

Taxonomy

Releasing artists' books from the topical constraints of critiquing the art market itself, artists are free to use their books to engage with any number of politics and institutions, including medicine. As well, the fracturing definitions of what is or is not considered an artist's book have led to a proliferation of overlapping categories for artists to situate themselves within while grappling with topics of illness and disability. What follows is a brief taxonomy of medically oriented artistic books for readers to help organize the vast array of printed matter they may come across.

An *illustrated book* is one that incorporates artistically rendered images alongside another's authored text. While the techniques used to make the images may be the same ones that printmakers use to make artists' books, the purpose of the book may be more commercial or educational, rather than an original piece of art in its own right.[14] Medical examples of this

13 Drucker, *The Century of Artists' Books*, 94.
14 Ibid., 5.

medium include historical anatomical treatises like the Andreas Vesalius' (1514–1564) preeminent book of anatomy, *De humani corporis fabrica* (1543). *Livre d'artist* or *deluxe editions* could also fall under the category of illustrated books because they are all defined as collaboration between printmakers, authors, and publishers rather than all of these roles falling to a single person as is typical of artists' books. A livre d'artist is a "limited edition, handmade book combining original prints with the artist often supervising the production of the book and collaborating with the author of the text."[15] William Blake, having apprenticed and made a career for himself as an engraver, was often commissioned to provide illustrations for medical textbooks. For example, Blake was hired to engrave plates for the English edition of Johann Caspar Lavater's *Essays on Physiognomy* (1789). This example shows how overlapping the categories of "art" and "illustration" can be even within a single person's practice, while also further entangling the connections between artists and the dissemination of medical thought.

Perhaps the closest format to the Fluxus artists' books of the 1970s is what we now refer to as *zines*, short for magazines. The significance of zines draws from their uncensored expression, collage aesthetic, quick printing, and potential for broad distribution in unnumbered, serial editions. Zines began and continue to be used as activist publishing because of their inexpensive photocopy printing and immediacy of thought within subcultures and political groups. Zines utilize hand-drawn or collaged content while keeping the form rather consistent: a single softcover folio, editioned by Xerox or Risograph copiers, and bound using a pamphlet stitch or staples. Artists' books can be quite different in this regard, where the form itself is highly implicated in the overall meaning of the book.

Medical zines tend to strike a balance between education, entertainment, and activism, and are typically created by and for particular patient communities. Examples of these publications include *Strip AIDS* (1987) out of the UK or *Diseased Pariah News* (1990–1999), which were created to educate readers about HIV/AIDS, safer sex practices, and give advice on living well with illness. Another notable publication is the *Toomeyville*

15 Jet Marie Prendeville, "Livres d'artistes: 1918 to 2000: A Very Special Collection," *The Flyleaf* 56, no. 1 (2009): 5.

Gazette, whose long run (1955–1998) crowdsourced know-how for helping disabled people live more independently, like how to alter common household objects to conform with impaired bodies, product reviews, job postings, and articles about what it is like to live and work with impairments. The general purpose of these and other illness and disability zines is to connect a dispersed community around their common experiences. Although none of these publications would be considered artists' books, they did print art, creative writing, and comics submitted by their subscribers.

Close relatives to medical zines are *illness comics* and the longer-format *Graphic Medicine* publications, otherwise known as *Graphic Pathographies*. The familiar narrative layout of comic cells, inclusion of humor, and complexity of deeply personal portrayals of life possible between text and image make this book form particularly prevalent within patient groups and medical education. Like artists' books, illness comics emphasize the personal and social impacts of living with a diagnosis or disability, typically written from the first-person perspective. Giving authority to patients to define their own lived experiences in these accessible, graphic formats "could therefore be seen as seizing power away from the 'official' iconography that informs society's notion of an illness."[16] However, a growing number of how-to workshops and graphic novel publications specifically geared toward medical professionals are rapidly expanding this artistic book genre. Even within the professional's perspective, these works tend to highlight the personal and psychological tolls of operating within medical systems.

The overlap between artists' books and illness comics can be so vast that it is often the writer-makers themselves that make the final distinction. For example, artist Jenny Lin states that she made two versions of her book, *Skinny Leg* (2012), which portrays and narrates her years-long trauma and recovery after being run over by a truck (see Figure 2.1). One version of *Skinny Leg* digitally reproduces her drawings and text into a single folded and stapled folio, which Lin categorizes as a graphic novel. The other version of *Skinny Leg* is screen printed by Lin, and constructed by hand with

16 Ian C. M. Williams, "Graphic Medicine: The Portrayal of Illness in Underground and Autobiographical Comics," in *Medicine, Health and the Arts: Approaches to Medical Humanities*, eds. Victoria Bates, Alan Bleakley, and Sam Goodman (London: Routledge, 2013), 74.

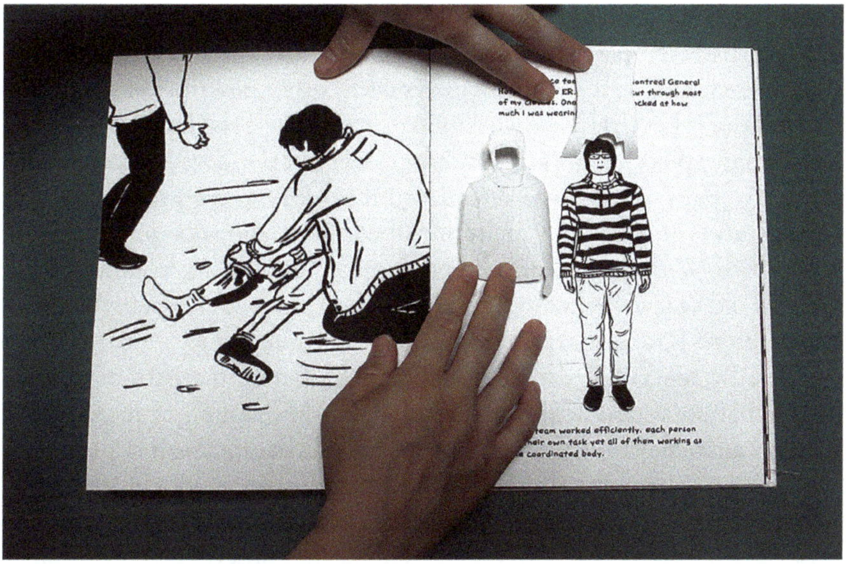

Figure 2.1: Jenny Lin, *Skinny Leg*, Silkscreen, 10″ × 7.5″, 2012. Image courtesy of the artist. <http://jenny-lin.ca/skinny.html>

pop-ups, foldouts, and bound within a hardcover.[17] Lin identifies this version of her narrative as an artist's book because the handcrafted elements of bookness propel the conceptual content of living with a traumatic injury.

This is not to say that the inclusion of handcrafted and multi-sensory elements are always indicative of an artist's book. Anatomical treatises throughout the Renaissance and beyond frequently included flaps to organize and reveal the structures of the human body, including Vesalius' *De fabrica*. A reader could lift off the flesh of the printed figure and, organ by organ, move through the layers of anatomy. In addition to portraying the third dimension within the flat plane of a book, flaps could also be employed to show change over time within the economy of a single page. Edward Tuson's book of midwifery, *Myology* (1828), employs flaps to display how the pregnant body changes throughout gestation, the movement of the fetus through the birth canal, and even the stages of a C-section

17 To see more of Lin's work, visit her website: <http://jenny-lin.ca/skinny.html>

procedure. One Lancet review of *Myology* from 1829 reads, "In the study of these dissected plates, the sense of touch is exercised as well as that of sight; hence their vast superiority over every other description of graphic illustration."[18] Because these works were conceived of as education material rather than a piece of fine art, they would not be considered artists' books. The use of flaps were a dimensional, multi-sensory, and temporal method of illustrating and teaching anatomy, albeit quite laborious and expensive to produce. With the inventions of automated publishing techniques, the flaps fell out of favor in anatomy textbooks and are today generally reserved for children's books or artists' books like Lin's *Skinny Leg.*

Finally, one could also draw a distinction between artists' books and books that are purely sculptural, that is, books that are not meant to be read because they do not contain text, do not have navigable pages, are static objects that appear as books, or are sculptures made out of books. Attempts have been made to categorize book sculptures under terms like *book works* or *art as book*,[19] but "artist's book" has prevailed as the popular term for even this kind of work. Tangy Duff's *Cryobook Archives* (2010–present) are an example of sculptural book works that, while their pages are blank and cannot be touched by their audience because they exist in a frozen cryochamber, are still considered artists' books because of their conceptual linkages between books and bodies. These works are investigated in much closer detail in the next chapter.

In spite of the usefulness of a taxonomy to orient a study of artists' books on illness, the issue of what artists' book are and how they intersect with medicine and the body is hardly settled—and that's a good thing. As soon as a medium attains a set definition, it limits the kinds of exploration of materials and forms possible. Turbulent categorizations promote experimentation and keep modes of expression lively and applicable to the unique perspective of each maker, rather than conforming creation to an archetype.

18 Westminster Medical Society, "Supplement to Myology," *The Lancet* 11, no. 280 (January 1829): 468.

19 Klima, *Artists Books*, 25.

Collecting Artists' Books

Artists' books are attractive to medical archives because they offer an experience very different to a typical illness memoir. Poetic, sensory, and generally able to be read within a single sitting, this medium provides a means to engage with illness narratives within an already over-booked medical curriculum. The accessible nature of creating an artist's book, especially compared to writing and publishing a memoir, also has the potential to diversify the voices represented in library collections. Artists' books enable a breadth of artistic illness expression that does not rely on narrative "completeness" or text at all, for that matter. For example, the head of artist's book acquisitions for the Wellcome Trust in London, Melanie Grant, states in our interview that the reason they began collecting artists' books in 2016 was to make space "for the ways in which people were expressing themselves creatively, and talking about their lived experience that wasn't necessarily in a traditional kind of memoir."[20] Finally, the stability of a book object lends permanence and authority to self-published narratives, while other forms of emergent narratives like social media or blog posts can be quickly buried. Within archival, tangible formats, artists' books demonstrate that the lasting impact of illness narratives is not only constituted by what the author says but also the very medium through which we read them.

Cataloging artists' books enables more women to occupy shelf space in medical and academic institutions, whose holdings traditionally privilege white male perspectives.[21] In our interview, Miller expresses her interest in collecting artists' books by women, who also tend to create the majority of artists' books on topics of medicine and illness. Perhaps this is no coincidence. In a situation where one has very little control over the most profound matters of one's life, like the diagnosis and treatment of cancer, compounded within an institution that has historically excluded women

20 Melanie Grant, interview by Darian Goldin Stahl, March 27, 2019.

21 Claire Hooker and Estelle Noonan, "Medical Humanities as Expressive of Western Culture," *Medical Humanities* 37, no. 2 (2011): 83.

from position of authority, it may be no wonder that women seek out an authoritative medium like artists' books to express these experiences. Artists' books may also be particularly salient for women due to their history of circumventing male-dominated gallery and publishing systems, the bodily closeness and intimacy the medium provides, and the inclusivity of typically women's media like sewing, scrapbooking, or journaling.[22]

Artists' books are also an avenue to decolonize perspectives on illness within university archives. The narrow confines of peer-reviewed commercial publishing disproportionately neglect BIPOC (Black, Indigenous, and People of Color) writers,[23] despite well-documented evidence that membership to racial minority communities negatively impacts health outcomes.[24] To counter this representational gap, Grant states that library curators must constantly question whose voices are missing within their holdings, "and then try and figure out where those voices are, and start to bring them into our collections."[25] Another librarian seeking equitable archives is Jane Ann Carlin at the University of Puget Sound, who attempts to decolonize the archives by specifically collecting artists' books by BIPOC authors for its Race and Pedagogy Institute. Carlin states that "artists' books offer the library the opportunity to build collections that represent distinct points of view and contribute new voices to scholarly discussions."[26]

Although artists' books are known as a "democratic medium" because of their low barriers of entry, librarians must nevertheless be vigilant to the

22 Stella Bolaki, "The Material Power of Artists' Books: How Books Can Speak about Illness and Care," in *Prescriptions: Artists' Books on Wellbeing and Medicine*, eds. Stella Bolaki and Egidija Ciricaite (London: Natrix Natrix Press, 2017), 6.

23 Amos Paul Kennedy Jr., "Social Book Building," in *Talking the Boundless Book: Art, Language, and the Book Arts*, ed. Charles Alexander (Minneapolis: Minnesota Center for Book Arts, 1995), 51.

24 Susan Merrill Squier, "Beyond Nescience: The Intersectional Insights of Health Humanities," *Perspectives in Biology and Medicine* 50, no. 3 (2007): 345, Project Muse.

25 Grant, interview.

26 Jane Anne Carlin, "Artists' Books as Catalysts for Social Change," *Art Libraries Journal* 44, no. 1 (2019): 2.

ways institutional archives stubbornly uphold Western settler perspectives.[27] Forming equitable collections is an ongoing practice of interrogating who makes archives, who is included in the holdings, who has access to holdings, and who does not. University archives are mostly out of reach to the general public or are not well equipped for accommodating people with impairments. Rarely are artists' books accompanied by accessibility measures like audio recitations, visual descriptions, or even images of the books on internet catalogs. While there are examples of artists who specifically seek out medical institutions to hold their artists' books on illness in order to influence new generations of doctors, like artist Martha Hall who is featured in Chapter 5, it would be a disservice to the outreaching potential of these works to constrain them to strictly professionalized contexts. With regard to who has access to view artists' books like Hall's, it is also worth scrutinizing the ways archives exclude certain illness or disability populations at the same time they attempt to represent them.

For researchers like me who already possess substantial privileges to conduct fieldwork within institutional spaces, the process of viewing archived artists' books was not straightforward. At the University of Kent, I had to attain a Visiting Scholar title with library access, identify and contact the correct librarian, choose only ten books to view per day from limited images on the online catalog (though any imagery at all is more than most catalogs), find the small viewing room within the sprawling library, leave all of my belongings in a locker, and finish looking at the books within a predetermined timeframe. Although making artists' books has a high level of accessibility, viewing them presents what may be insurmountable hurdles for most. For her part, the special collections librarian at the University of Kent, Joanna Baines, acknowledges that these artists' books have untapped potential to positively impact people who would not be able or willing to go through the effort to visit these books in person.[28] She hopes to enact future programming in which artists' books will be taken into hospitals

27 For further dialogue on the topic of decolonizing archives, see: Stephanie Springgay, Anise Truman, and Sara MacLean, "Socially Engaged Art, Experimental Pedagogies, and Anarchiving as Research-Creation," *Qualitative Inquiry* 5, no. 1 (2019): 1–11.

28 Joanna Baines, interview by Darian Goldin Stahl, January 31, 2019.

and clinics, where they can fulfill Hall's wish "to touch the hearts of people who themselves are battling cancer or a life-threatening disease."[29]

On the other hand, it may be difficult to balance the desire for wide and frequent public access to these books with the archive's mandate for preservation. This is especially true for artists' books whose delicate materiality may not fall within a book restorer's typical repertoire. A workaround to broaden public access to artists' books is to provide more detailed photographs of every page and searchable keyword catalogs. However, the variable size, shape, and navigation of each artist's books makes effectively photographing them particularly challenging.[30] As well, the feel, weight, smell, temporality, and other sensory information that make up a large portion of the book's overall meaning is lost. I propose that video walkthroughs of the books that include audio recitation, captions, and visual descriptions are the most accessible and faithful digital format for artists' books, with full acknowledgment of the impossibility (or unwillingness) of hosting such large format files on university servers.

Artists' books demand to be touched in order to fulfill their pedagogical purpose. Democratizing this access may mean letting go of standards of pristineness and prioritizing how these books can be made present and useful in the present tense, rather than perfectly preserving them in perpetuity. As artists' books continue to be collected by university archives, the types of book objects considered archivable will also need to expand significantly. If only artists' books that adhere to comfortable codex forms, fit on a shelf, or are constructed with materials that will not change over time will be collected, then the archive will inevitably limit creativity and exclude certain sensory knowledges.

It is also worth cautioning that the institutionalization of artists' books, including their widening appeal in medical library special collections, may consequently limit the topics and uncensored criticality provoked within their pages. How much critique is the medical library willing to accept against its own institution? On the other hand, the pressure to curb one's

29 Martha Hall, "Artist Statement," in *Holding In, Holding On: Artist's Books by Martha A. Hall*, eds. Martha Hall and Martin Antoinette (Northampton: Mortimer Rare Book Room, Smith College, 2003).

30 Egidija Ciricaite, "On Photographing Artist's Books," *Journal of Medical Humanities* 41, (2020): 81.

critical experiences of medical systems in favor of securing an acquisition could also perpetuate a sense of moral compromise and loss of control they felt as patients in the first place. This is difficult terrain to navigate, especially considering the economic constraints against sustainable arts practices that are still recovering from the 2008 recession and will continue to face hardships from the fallout of Covid-19. In my view, supporting artists is the top priority. Librarians must therefore advocate for paying for works that add meaning to medicine, even if the works take a critical stance. Also, if artists choose to compromise or censor their ideas to gain access to medical spaces, achieving any representation in the stacks may ultimately pave the way for more subversive works in the future.

One final concern for the librarians is how to justify the value of particular artists' books given tightening budget restrictions. Should funds be diverted to acquiring artists' books based on artistic merit, to represent a particular illness, provide a missing perspective, diversify holdings, or some other criteria? For arts-based researchers like Leavy, academic institutions should acquire works not based on the level of craft achieved, but on the *usefulness* of the artworks for "communicating information about the experiences associated with differences, diversity, and prejudice."[31] The librarians I spoke with agree. The value they find in these books is not necessarily based on how "good" they are in an aesthetic sense, but if and how they fill gaps in knowledge within the library's collection. Grant attests, "[I]f an artist's book is saying something important, that's maybe not being said somewhere else, even if it's not necessarily the most successful artists' book you will come across, then it still has some value to us." The aim of these collections for medical learning places priority on the breadth of illness perspectives over subjective standards of aesthetics.

On the other hand, if artists' books on illness are to be taken seriously as objects worth collecting and viewing, then it is important that they contain sufficient artistic merit to attract and engage the reader and not simply appreciated that they were created at all. If the works are not aesthetically engaging, then they risk being viewed as user-friendly helpers to the more

31 Patricia Leavy, *Method Meets Art: Arts-Based Research Practice* (New York City: Guilford Press, 2015), 24.

rigorous genre of illness memoirs rather than powerhouses of sensory expressions in their own right. These artists' books must be alluring enough to entice audiences inside and outside of medical contexts if they are to enact challenges to dominant (mis-)conceptions of illness.

Conclusion

Printed matter on illness spans a breadth of formats categorized as "books," each with their own standards of bookness, histories, and strategies to communicate the story within. Artists' books' nebulous and evolving definition has evaded concrete standards for what could or could not fall under this umbrella term. The border crossing medium thus remains dynamic to fit the needs of each maker to represent themselves with fidelity—a modal flexibility that becomes all the more important to encourage representation from a full range of perspectives and abilities.

Like all activist art, there is debate on the effectiveness of artwork to instigate meaningful change if it remains unnoticed by those who hold the most power. Until very recently, artists' books, graphic novels, and zines were not circulated within medical education and thus had little influence on those populations.[32] However, with the rapid rise of printed matter on illness from libraries and special collections, artists' books are beginning to find an audience *within* medical institutions. Heroic efforts from individual librarians are meeting the call to broaden what can and ought to be held within their institutions, acknowledging the ongoing history of exclusionary acquisition practices and privileged viewing spaces of academic libraries. While this chapter outlines some critiques of accessibility to meaningfully engage with artists' books on illness and disability for many with lived experiences of those same topics, the next chapter takes a closer look at the critiques against the legacies of Western medical culture within the books themselves.

32 Johanna Drucker, "Bound to Speak: Accounts of Illness in Artists' Books," *Journal of Medical Humanities* 41, no. 1 (2020): 86.

CHAPTER 3

The Artist's Challenge to Medical Paradigms

Introduction

The progress of medicine can be seen through its images: from the drawn, engraved, or etched representations of the body printed and bound into tomes by collaborating anatomists and artists, to the digitally stacked slices of biomedical scans produced by penetrating waves of magnetic resonance. These visualizations not only show us the hidden depths of our own anatomies but also how Western medicine has enduringly arranged the structures of body into paginated layers. In tandem with the advancement of science, evermore finely tuned and efficient printmaking techniques have evolved to disseminate medical thinking throughout the centuries.

Even though historical books on anatomy and pathology are not considered artists' books, their printing techniques and artistry are nevertheless intertwined with the development of the visual culture of medicine that influences artists' books on illness today. On the other hand, even though artists' books are not presenting medical knowledge per se, they employ the authority of medical illustration to flip the hierarchy between medical conceptualizations of disease and the health knowledge acquired through living with illness. A close examination of the intersections of medical treatises and artists' books demonstrates how those who capitalize on the format of books as icons of knowledge seize authority over the bodies printed between their covers.

To exemplify the longitudinal links between medical books and contemporary artists' books, I will focus on two main artworks, *The Gynecologist* (1989) by Joan Lyons and the *Cryobook Archives* (2010–present) by Tagny Duff. These two works in particular also demonstrate the power of artistic appropriation as a tool to focus renewed attention on the underlying themes and cultural significance of medical representations of the body. Both *The Gynecologist* and *Cryobook Archives* take up historical anatomical images and re-present them with a contemporary lens in order to sensitize readers to persistently harmful cultural paradigms, such as paternalism, skin-tone bias, and patient objectification. By reprinting centuries-old illustrations or replicating bygone anatomical bookmaking practices, these artists exhibit and then critique the long arc of influence between those with medical power and those seeking healing. Finally, I will introduce the critical health humanities as a space to mobilize artists' books and foster *parallaxic practice*, or the multimodal and interdisciplinary collaboration design of research, analysis, and pedagogy.[1]

Phenomenology, and in particular feminist phenomenology, provides a framework to analyze the power dynamics of printing bodies. Phenomenology attempts to expose and critique the taken-for-granted assumptions that influence everyday life, and feminist phenomenology concentrates a particular lens on how "marginalization, invisibility, nonnormativity, and oppression"[2] influence such everyday occurrences. Within the topic of medicine, feminist phenomenology is particularly relevant to understand illness experiences of women and People of Color, whose voices have been historically excluded from positions of medical power and whose marginalization still reverberates throughout the institution. This chapter thus draws a jagged line across the knotty sticking points of medical history that contemporary artists feel compelled to unveil and address. In an effort to scrutinize patriarchal and colonial lineages that still influence medical decisions today, artists grasp the power of the printed page for themselves and enter underrepresented voices into critical

1 Pauline Sameshima, Patricia Maarhuis, and Sean Wiebe, *Parallaxic Practice: Multimodal Interdisciplinary Pedagogical Research Design* (Wilmington: Vernon Press, 2019), 1.

2 Lisa Folkmarson Käll and Kirstin Zeiler, "Why Feminist Phenomenology and Medicine?," in *Feminist Phenomenology and Medicine*, eds. Lisa Folkmarson Käll and Kirstin Zeiler (Albany: SUNY Press, 2014), 8.

and feminist health humanities dialogues. As phenomenological engagements with artists' books articulate experiences within healthcare systems from marginalized patients, the particular combination of image, text, and materiality makes otherness tangible and heard.

Artists' Books as a Critique of the Cultural Paradigms of Medicine

The art of medicine has two facets. First is the scientific half, which sets as its very foundation a practice of self-critique and evolution. Laboratory medicine continuously tests assumptions, standards, and methods to achieve evermore precise and effective treatments. The other half is the practice of medicine within culture, where societal norms, laws, and politics influence how patients receive care. While scientific medicine can achieve rapid change with new technological innovations, the culture of medicine is much slower to evolve. Artists working in this context attempt to promote a practice of critique, perhaps more akin to the reflexive practices of scientific medicine, toward the hegemonic paradigms of Western medical culture.

Given their activist origins, it is no surprise that artists' books are still today conceived of as grassroots endeavors to disseminate political ideas and influence social consciousness—and medicine is not exempt from a critical review. One way artists use the influence of their book creations to advocate for better patient care is by appropriating the medical images of the past and reprinting them with contemporary ethics, which demonstrates just how sticky certain discriminatory cultural norms remain. Artists who re-present medical illustrations according to their own world view are performing a critique of the institution of medicine that has historically excluded women, People of Color, the disabled, and other marginalized populations until very recently. By making and disseminating artists' books on this topic, space then opens for a productive reexamination of such Western medical paradigms.

Joan Lyons: The Gynecologist (1989)

Joan Lyons' *The Gynecologist* (1989) is a single folio, soft cover artist's book whose relatively simple form and staple binding contrast with the depth of conceptual complexities within (see Figure 3.1). Using black and white ink printed with offset lithography on tan paper, Lyons appropriates and reprints images of women's bodies, organs, and gynecological medical devices from landmark anatomical publications over the past 500 years. Whole figures appear on the left-hand side of the page spreads, and patterned disembodied organs float like uncanny wallpaper behind text boxes printed on the right-hand pages. The text transcribes an interview with a woman who recounts years of contentious interactions with her gynecologist as he pressures her to have a hysterectomy. Printed together, the peculiar anatomical illustrations set against the patient's own voice highlight historical misconceptions of female anatomy and the pressures women continue to face to submit to gynecological surgeries with unclear long-term consequences. *The Gynecologist* is thus emblematic of patriarchal and paternalistic paradigms that insidiously permeate medical culture.

The proliferation of medical imagery in the twentieth century, such as x-rays and affordable anatomical atlases, alongside accessible copy printing like the Xerox, practically invites artists to appropriate these representations of the body and explore their more unsettling implications. Women in particular pick up and re-present these old anatomical illustrations because, as historian Ludmilla Jordanova explains, "they feel that the theories and practices of medicine have exercised disproportionate power over women's bodies; they want to re-form the representations of the female body in order to affirm the value of women as subjects (including artistic ones)."[3] Within the space of their artists' books, women are empowered to redress the lack of their own first-person perspectives in the formation of healthcare knowledge about them.

3 Deanna Petherbridge and Ludmilla Jordanova, *The Quick and the Dead: Artists and Anatomy* (Manchester: Cornerhouse Publications, 1997), 112.

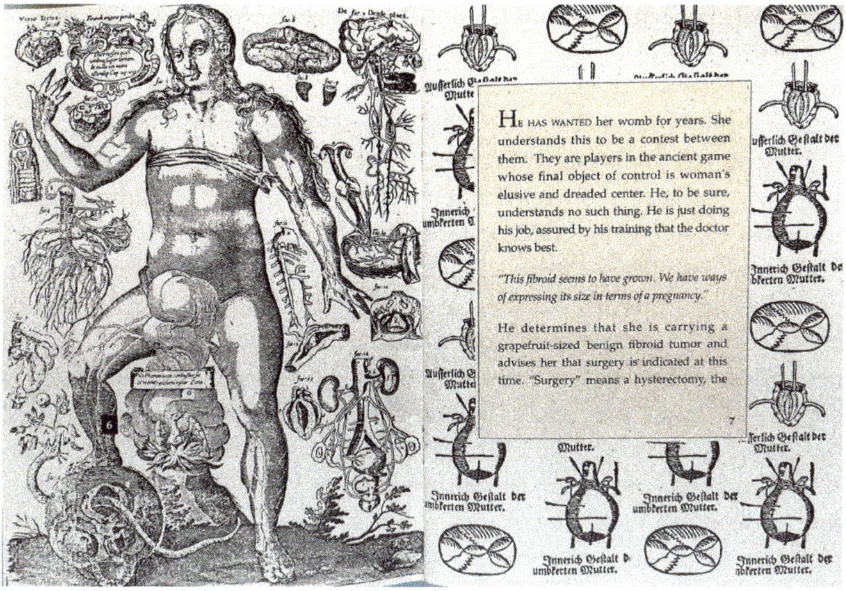

Figure 3.1: Joan Lyons, *The Gynecologist*, Offset lithography, 8.5″ × 6″, 1989.

The women's bodies reprinted within *The Gynecologist* reach back into the 1500s and portray an ornate visual culture that is quite different from today's standard of austere and objective medical illustration. The Renaissance was a time when art, science, religion, and philosophy could exist together rather than in separated fields, therefore it was commonplace for anatomical illustrations to include grander visual allegories.[4] For example, anatomical depictions of women's bodies would often double as biblical allegories for Eve. The first visual trope of the anatomical Eve appropriated and reprinted in *The Gynecologist* is by the German anatomist Johann Remmelin (1583–1632), whose illustrations were then engraved by Lucas Kilian (1579–1637) for the book, *Catoptrum microcosmicum*, first officially published in 1619 (see Figure 3.1). This dense image portrays a snake with an apple tree branch in its mouth slithering through a skull under

4 Martin Kemp, "Foreword," in *The Physician's Art,* eds. Julie Hansen and Suzanne Porter (Durham: Duke University Press, 1999), 14.

Eve's foot. In the background, a phoenix is erupting from a volcano, the ash of which wafts into the foreground to cover Eve's genitals. References to Genesis, Greek mythology, *memento mori*, and the promise of life after death present an eccentric array of allegories in this anatomical image.

Although this is perhaps the most ornate Eve figure reprinted within *The Gynecologist*, it is certainly not the last. Flipping through the illustrations that span so many centuries, it strikes the reader how stylistically and positionally similar the female figures remain. I take this homogeneity to exemplify how typical it was for anatomists, illustrators, engravers, and publishers to appropriate and copy one another. Publishers cut costs by copying previous work rather than commissioning new illustrations. Indeed, exact copies of Vesalius' plates (also included in *The Gynecologist*) can be found again and again in anatomical treatises, including Remmelin's aforementioned treatise. Aside from the desire to pirate Vesalius and his illustrator Jan Stephan van Calcar's extraordinarily popular imagery, including the plates, portraits, and anatomical notions of forebears was also a method of paying homage to a lineage of medical thinkers. Vesalius himself faced some professional backlash for *de Fabrica* when he broke with conventions to exclude most of the, albeit false, conventions of Galenic anatomy established and upheld for the thirteen centuries prior. Ideas of how the body looks and works become engrained as medical fact when the same plates are reprinted over and over, each new publisher depending on the accuracy of the former, even when new scientific discoveries prove those images to be inaccurate. Although anatomy is considered a science, the depiction of medicalized bodies would seem to be heavily influenced by the glacially paced culture in which they are printed. This explains why the same tropes and misinformation of female anatomy appear again and again—effectively cementing them into the visual culture of medicine.

By reprinting images of female genitalia from 500 years of medical illustration, Lyons shows how biased or even false anatomical representations become standard thinking. For example, the idea that the female reproductive organs are more or less undescended, internal penises was illustrated in the Renaissance and severely influenced how they were represented for centuries—as Lyons displays throughout her artist's book. A phallic bias was able to take root because the male body was understood as the standard, representative body. While male anatomical illustrations depicted all states of exposed musculature, veins, viscera, and ossification, depictions of female anatomy were typically reserved only for the structures that deviated from male anatomy: the primary and secondary sex organs. Even within sex organ illustrations, female structures and fluids were conceptualized as derivative of those of males, so that maleness could be understood as universal and femaleness as stunted or deviant.[5] The phallic uteruses reprinted throughout Lyon's pages are meant to exemplify how patriarchy can hinder accurate female anatomical knowledge.

Page after page, Lyons reproduces female anatomical figures that follow a common stylization where the female subject's faces and breasts remain alluring and unscarred by the anatomist's scalpel, while their abdomens are cut open to reveal either a fetus or hollow gut cavity awaiting to be filled. This visual trope often takes center stage within the title pages of many anatomy treatises: a nude female figure laying on the dissection table at the center of an anatomy theater, breasts and face intact, abdomen flayed open, and surrounded by crowds of well-dressed men. Lyons demonstrates the staying power of this particular composition as she reprints the title page of Vesalius' *Epitome* (1540) all the way to photographic reproductions like "Howard Atwood Kelly About to Operate" (1897) and the advertisement for surgical supplies, *Great Moments in Medicine* (1945), by Lejaren a Hiller. This depiction of women in anatomical illustrations tacitly upholds the idea that a woman's role in medicine is, at most, to be an object of study and never of medical authority. Given that women were generally shunned from attaining medical degrees until the 1960s, it may be no wonder that this composition held fast as one of the quintessential visual representations for the art of practicing medicine.

This is not to say that enormous strides toward gender equality have bypassed the practice of medicine but to underscore how the lasting effects of a medical institution that was established without women in positions of authority can be witnessed in its visual culture. Lyons' appropriation and reprinting of medical images portray such a stymied development of female anatomical knowledge. Although it may be unfair to judge the

5 Petherbridge and Jordanova, *The Quick and the Dead*, 63.

practices of the past with contemporary standards of medical ethics, artists feel compelled to redress these images precisely because their affects are still felt within the examination room today.

In the afterword of *The Gynecologist*, Lyons explains that "while modern medical practice has removed the horns from its anatomical description of the uterus and no longer insists on a phallic representation of female genitalia, the mythic elements that informed these representations lives on in the still largely patriarchal practice of gynecology."[6] A preponderance of focus on male anatomy has led to rippling detrimental effects to women's healthcare. For example, new models of female sexual organs are still being refined because "typical textbook descriptions of the clitoris lack detail and include inaccuracies."[7] A survey of anatomical textbooks from the twentieth century by O'Connell et al. found that later editions of the same medical textbooks even deleted descriptive text of the clitoris—willfully perpetuating the ignorance of female anatomy due to social biases. As surgery depends on the accurate illustration and description of anatomy, omissions such as this have serious consequences for urology, pelvic, and gynecology patients.

In an effort to include women's voices rather than solely their inert bodies in healthcare discourses, Lyons transcribes an interview with a woman who felt coerced by her physician to undergo a hysterectomy. Lyons likens their debate to two "players in the ancient game whose final object of control is the woman's elusive and dreaded center."[8] In the course of the artist's book, we read the physician pressure his patient by instilling fears that her benign uterine fibroid may become cancerous in the future, the higher risks of surgical complications and blood loss if she decides to wait, and even potentially contracting AIDS through multiple blood transfusions. He also attempts to bate her with the promise of a permanent form of birth control and no longer having menstruation cycles so she can perform at top levels "like [his] other patients who are important people—lawyers," and "be like everybody else."[9] The pressure tactics and belittlement of the

6 Joan Lyons, *The Gynecologist* (Rochester: The Visual Studies Workshop, 1989), 23.

7 Helen E. O'Connell, Kalavampara V. Sanjeevan, and John M. Huston, "Anatomy of the Clitoris," *Journal of Urology* 179 (2005): 1189.

8 Lyons, *The Gynecologist*, 7.

9 Ibid., 19.

narrator's chosen career as an artist do not deter her, and she continues to ask questions that champion her long-term health outcomes from an elective total removal of her hormone-producing organs, rather than submit to medical paternalism.

At the publication of *The Gynecologist* in 1989, hysterectomies were (and still are) the "second most frequently performed major surgical procedure among reproductive-aged women in the United States," and one in four women had a hysterectomy by the time they reached 60 years of age.[10] Over thirty years later, medical opinion is beginning to change on the high prevalence of this major surgery. The long-term consequences of hysterectomies, including "fracture risk, pelvic floor dysfunction, all-cause mortality, cardiovascular disease, and neurologic function," as well as the mood-boosting effects of retaining one's androgen-producing organs, may outweigh the risks presented by benign uterine fibroids.[11] In hindsight, it seems the concerns presented by Lyons' interview subject were perfectly valid and prudent.

Engaging with this artist's book, I am most struck by the juxtaposition of inaccurate historical depictions of female anatomy and illustrations of submissive women's bodies set against an inquisitive woman's voice who appears to be a fierce self-advocate. The tension between the text and images exemplifies how much we still do not know about women's health, and the immense pressure many patients feel when questioning medical authority. In printing a private exchange between doctor and patient in a public format, others may incorporate similar sentiments of medical hierarchies they too have experienced into the meaning of this book, while also exemplifying how one may seize back some authority over their medical decisions by asking follow-up questions.

The influence of the collaboration between Lyons and her anonymous interviewee in *The Gynecologist* to promote women's health demonstrates a critical and feminist phenomenology. Critical in its activist motivations

10 Lisa A. Lepine et al., "Hysterectomy Surveillance—United States. 1980–1993," MMWR Surveillance Summaries, Centers for Disease Control, last modified September 19, 1998, <https://www.cdc.gov/mmwr/preview/mmwrhtml/00048898.htm>.

11 Elizabeth A. Stewart, Lynne T. Shuster, and Walter A Rocca, "Reassessing Hysterectomy," *Minnesota Medicine* 95, no. 3 (March 2012): 36–39.

and feminist in its subject matter, this artist's book unveils the biased history of a medicine system that has always exerted disproportionate power over women's bodies. Although *The Gynecologist* represents the experiences of one woman, the inclusion of imagery from over 500 years of medicine demonstrates that her feelings of diminished authority are not just common, but systemic to Western medical culture. A phenomenological intertwining of meaning between the maker to readers of *The Gynecologist* shows us that, once medical paternalism has been exposed in the otherwise private space of the clinic, "the capacity to move from the singularity of the standard first-person narrative to an account that seeks to identify and analyze generalities and typical features of the experience as such, … resides within and intersects with the broader lifeworld."[12] Once the dynamics of text and image solidify what medical paternalism can look like, it may then be extrapolated to the readers' individual situations and productively countered within their own physician interactions.

To propel the activist feminist message of this book, Lyons editioned this work to the high number of 800, which allows it to have a relatively low purchase price. This decision aligns with the "democratic multiple" model of artists' books for a wide distribution, which seeks to "inform women and thus give them back, if not control over their own bodies, at least support for negotiating rather than submitting to medical authority."[13] While the artist's book does not reveal whether the patient does ultimately receive a hysterectomy, it is clear her resilient self-advocacy in the midst of such medical pressures led her to feel more informed and at ease with this decision.

Tagny Duff: Cryobook Archives

Like Lyons, artist Tagny Duff positions her artist's books as a reexamination and critique of the dominant power of medicine over the patient's

12 Linda Fisher, "The Illness Experience: A Feminist Phenomenological Perspective," in *Feminist Phenomenology and Medicine*, eds. Lisa Folkmarson Käll and Kirstin Zeiler (Albany: SUNY Press, 2014), 34.

13 Joan Lyons, quoted by Johanna Drucker, *The Century of Artists' Books* (New York City: Granary Books, 1995), 293.

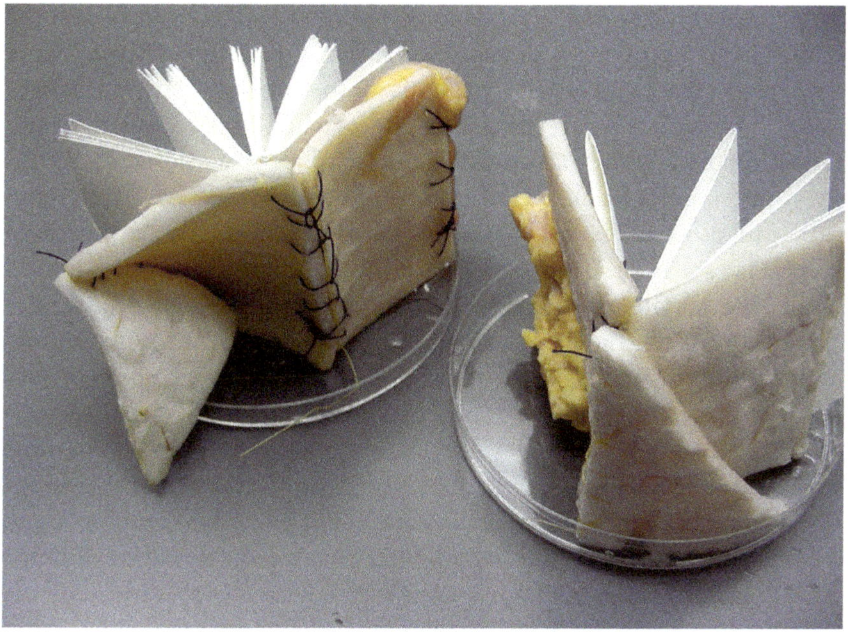

Figure 3.2: Tagny Duff, *Cryobook Archives*, Human and animal flesh and paper, 2010–present. Image courtesy of the artist. <http://tagnyduff.com/projects-current/cryobook-archives/>

body. However, rather than evidencing this hierarchy through internal anatomy, Duff focuses on the surface. The *Cryobook Archives* (2010–present) presents a series of four pocket-sized books that are bound in fleshy material (see Figure 3.2). Upon reading Duff's artist statement, the viewer is informed that the book covers are in fact made from animal and human flesh. The books contain folios of blank paper and are sewn to the cover using black surgical sutures. To keep the raw flesh from decaying, the books are housed in a wooden cabinet behind triple sealed glass, which sits upon a freezer unit that keeps the books in a cryogenic stasis at −80 °C.

Duff's work is meant to bring attention to the very real bodies behind the sterilized digital and illustrated images of anatomy, because "we often forget that information is made from physical bodies."[14] Although the human flesh was ethically donated to Duff's project from a living friend, she explains that these books are also meant to evoke historical practices of "grave robbing," or the unscrupulous and nonconsensual acquisition and dissection of cadavers for the education of medical professionals, as well as the contemporary black market trading of human tissue. Duff calls on us to consider the "status and instrumentalization of bodies in the pursuit of knowledge and information"[15] by presenting flesh excised from their original bodies and literally objectified into the iconic symbol of learning, books.

In contrast to ornate anatomical illustrations of Eve figures, brawny cadavers dancing through the Italian country, or skeletons posed next to exotic animals, the great advancements to anatomy and Western medicine were made, quite literally, on the backs the poor, the enslaved, and those subjected to capital punishment. Great Britain's Murder Act of 1752 stipulated that especially egregious murderers could be further sentenced to *anatomization*, that is, medical dissection. This decree was meant to satiate both the schools of anatomy's requests for fresh corpses to dissect and the government's interest in deterring crime by desecrating the criminal corpse and denying an intact Christian burial.[16] Although the images produced for medical treatises were expensive and grand affairs whose figures are often characterized as upper-class members of society or even holy figures, the origins of these cadavers belonged to those on the fringes of society over whom the medical institution could exert its total control.

Such is the case of the crimes and curious afterlife of William Burke (1792–1829), who engaged in grave robbing and the sale of these corpses to eager schools of anatomy in Edinburgh. When Burke and his accomplice were found to have murdered sixteen people over a two-year spree in order to sell the bodies for medical education, he was sentenced to

14 Tagny Duff, "Cryobook Archives_Tagny Duff," filmed February 7, 2011 at the Science Gallery, Dublin, video, 2:44, <http://tagnyduff.com/projects-current/cryobook-archives/>.

15 Tagny Duff, "Cryobook Archives," accessed November 4, 2020, <http://tagnyduff.com/projects-current/cryobook-archives/>.

16 Sarah Tarlow and Emma Battell Lowman, *Harnessing the Power of the Criminal Corpse* (London: Palgrave Macmillan, 2018), 84.

death by hanging and, in a kind of self-fulfilling prophecy, also sentenced to anatomization at the University of Edinburgh by anatomy professor Alexander Monro III.[17] Monro then used Burke's excised flesh to create at least two calling card holders (what we might deem today as business card holders) and, most pertinent for this analysis, a pocket book. This small, dark brown folder would have been used to carry loose papers and notes. It is imprinted with the gold leaf title, "Burke's Skin Pocket Book" on the front, the date of his execution on the back, and boasts loops for conveniently holding writing utensils. Monro's series of morbid objects made from Burke's leather hide takes the intersection of bookmaking and medical objectification to its most extreme.

The practice of turning human flesh into books, known as *anthropodermic bibliopegy*, while rare, was certainly not unheard of. In most cases, the deceased's flesh was used to bind books of their murderous crimes or cover copies of anatomical treatises. Megan Rosenbloom's publication on this topic, *Dark Archives* (2021), explains that nearly all cases of anthropodermic bibliopegy were commissioned and supplied by doctors. Access to copious amounts of human skin from dissections, learned men's popular hobby of collecting rare books, and the symbolic synchrony of binding books of anatomy with human flesh all merge to cultivate this practice amongst physicians in the eighteenth and nineteenth centuries.[18] Prestigious medical institutions often hold these books today, including Harvard's Houghton Library, the Historical Medical Library of the College of Physicians of Philadelphia, and Brown University, which even counts an anthropodermic copy of Vesalius' *de Fabrica* among its collection. One can find *Burke's Skin Pocket Book* still on display at the Surgeons' Hall Museums in Edinburgh, Scotland.

These morbid items became valuable collectables, which is one of the rationales behind such a practice. Another reason is to lend a certain authenticity and gravitas to an anatomical textbook. A final justification for turning human flesh into books is to continue one's corporeal punishment

17 Sarah Tarlow, "Curious Afterlives: The Enduring Appeal of the Criminal Corpse," *Mortality* 21, no. 3 (2018): 216.

18 Megan Rosenbloom, *Dark Archives: A Librarian's Investigation into the Science and History of Books Bound in Human Skin* (New York: Picador, 2021), 47.

long after death. The flayed bodies of England's worst criminals were put on display as "part of the public humiliation of murderers implemented to deter future criminals."[19] Dehumanizing corpses by transforming them into books performed a sort of posthumous justice upon those deemed unable to learn from their mistakes or seemingly felt little-to-no value for the sanctity of life.

Claiming authority over the fate of flesh intertwined capital punishment with medical practices, but Rosenbloom recounts one example of a criminal reclaiming his skin's destiny. Career criminal George Walton, held in a Massachusetts prison upon his death in 1837, requested that the two copies of his memoir be bound in his own flesh.[20] Fulfilling his wishes, the attending physician excised Walton's skin and sent it to a tanner and book binder. Though we don't know his true motivations, it seems Walton was attempting to subvert the lack of control over his imprisoned body by requesting the objectification of it himself. Of the two resulting books, titled *Narrative of the Life of James Allen, Alias George Walton, Alias Jonas Pierce, Alias James H. York, Alias Burley Grove the Highwayman* (1837), one was given to the attending physician and the other went to John Fenno—Walton's robbery and shooting victim who lived to serve as witness against him in court. Fenno's daughter ultimately donated the book to the Boston Athenaeum; but before the donation, Fenno's copy of the book, "according to family lore, was used to spank naughty children and frighten them into good behavior."[21] Although he claimed agency over the creation of his book-body, Walton's objectification nevertheless served as a deterrent for misdeeds just as the other criminals' books before him.

Historian Constance Classen relays that schoolmasters would routinely beat their students in order to make "what one learnt part of one's innermost bodily experience,"[22] as it was thought that the memory of the painful beating would cement the day's learning along with it. For Burke, Walton, and others like them, could there be a more fitting fate than having

19 Ibid., 121.

20 Ibid., 150.

21 Ibid., 154.

22 Constance Classen, *The Deepest Sense: A Cultural History of Touch* (Urbana: University of Illinois Press, 2012), 19.

their skin bound into the cover of a book—the iconic symbol of societal knowledge and authority that the criminals so disregarded in life? Certainly, a lessoned has been learned in the transformation from body to book.

In the immediate aftermath of Burke's crimes and sensational trial, Great Britain passed the Anatomy Act of 1832, which stipulated that *any* unclaimed corpse, not just those of criminals, could now be acquired by anatomy schools in order to undercut the black market for corpses. This act effectively shifted the cache of cadavers from executed criminals to the extremely poor: those who remained unclaimed in the morgue, whose family could not afford a burial, or the enslaved. In America and other European colonial establishments, this meant that the medical advancements were disproportionately built upon the bodies of People of Color.[23] For example, Harriet A. Washington documents in her book, *Medical Apartheid* (2006), that the so-called "Father Modern of Gynecology," J. Marion Sims (1813–1883), honed his experimental techniques on Black slaves who had no rights to resist. However, Sims "hid his subjects' race and even illustrated reports of experiments on Black slave women with illustrations of bourgeois white matrons."[24] An application of medical knowledge garnered from the exploitation of Black bodies for the benefit of white bodies could be made palatable by obscuring the identity that skin provides.

When Black people *were* portrayed in medical textbooks and print media in the sixteenth though twentieth centuries, they were often accompanied by racist stereotypes and negative connotations. In humoral medicine, madness was diagnosed as the overabundance of black bile, which had the ability to darken a person's soul along with their skin—indicating the totality and permanence of the humoral imbalance that ultimately pervaded one's outward appearance. This, along with the iconography of small black demons biting the heads or leaping from the mouths of the Mad, formed the commonplace association between Madness and Blackness.[25] The evolution of illustrating Madness culminated in the eighteenth century with

23 Richard Barnett, *The Sick Rose* (London: Thames and Hudson, 2014), 38–39.

24 Harriet A. Washington, *Medical Apartheid: The Dark History of Medical Experimentation on Black Americans from Colonial Times to the Present* (New York: Harlem Moon Broadway Books, 2006), 59.

25 Sander Gilman, *Seeing the Insane* (Lincoln: University of Nebraska Press, 1996), 2.

the publication of pseudoscientific phrenology and physiognomy textbooks, where dispositions and intelligence could be read through cranial shapes and facial features, respectively. The founder of phrenology Franz Joseph Gall (1758–1828) and his book, *On the Functions of the Brain and of Each of Its Parts* (English translation published in 1835), concluded that the facial features of those from African descent were most closely linked with criminality and mental illness. Backed by the power of medical and anatomical "findings," attributions of criminality and Madness could be foisted onto the Black identity by those who sought to justify their continued dehumanization, subjugation, and enslavement.

No anthropodermic books have been confirmed to be bound in Black skin, though they most likely exist and many are purported to be.[26] Current forensic technologies cannot definitively differentiate if these skin books originate from Black bodies, but we know the people who collected them were white. There are many examples of fraudulent flesh books that claim to be made of Black skin in order to make them more appealing for collectors, either by reinforcing our ideas of how People of Color are already dehumanized or appealing to those who would prefer to own a book made with Black skin. We do know there was rampant exploitation of Black bodies and cadavers by medical professionals that could have been sources of skin, and that it was common to take body parts from lynching victims as mementos.[27]

Due to systemic economic disparities and the standard practice of utilizing unclaimed bodies for medical education, Black people were at the highest risk of anatomization in many parts of America until the Uniform Anatomical Gift Act of 1968, which enabled the wide practice of consensual anatomical donation. However, "the legacy of this 'postmortem racism' survives in policies that continue to appropriate the bodies of 'friendless paupers' such as the homeless—a disproportionate number of whom are Black—for medical purposes."[28] Although the number of anatomized Black bodies outpaces the racial ratios of the United States, there continues to be

26 Rosenbloom, *Dark Archives*, 103.

27 Washington, *Medical Apartheid*, 136.

28 Ibid., 118.

a white bias within the illustrations of medical textbooks today. A recent survey found that the most common textbooks and anatomical atlases currently used in medical schools disproportionately portray light skin tones relative to population proportions, even though certain diseases, like skin cancer, can appear strikingly different on darker skin.[29] Therefore, "a lack of attention to race/ethnicity in case examples reinforces whiteness as the assumed norm,"[30] to the detriment of health outcomes experienced by People of Color.

The history of medicine's tumultuous authority over flesh is highlighted by Duff's *Cryobook Archive*. The human flesh in this work is not obscured nor its color altered, but is the raw focus of attention. Duff has chosen to retain a life-like vitality for this flesh rather than alter or preserve it through tanning procedures. The pallor and details of hair and freckles, as if it is still living atop the person who made it, lay bare the traces of a real human life. These one-of-a-kind books appeal to the idea that each person contains their own particular history and life experience. Duff means to preserve the notion that flesh remains a rightful site of humanity and identity by preserving this particular skin, as is, in a cryogenic book cabinet to evoke the idea of each individual as an everlasting archive.

Duff's work takes up anatomical practices of the past and returns it with new ethics of consent and reciprocity. Unlike previous examples of anthropodermic bibliopegy or forced anatomization, Duff attained full consent from a living donor whose flesh was excised during a cosmetic surgery. Although the viewer of these books is not permitted to take them out of cryogenic stasis to hold them, the visceral quality of the flesh covers, including their visible yellow fat and black suture binding, reaches out to the viewer to provoke an empathetic sense of pain. This intermingling of the person who donated their skin and the viewers' gut reactions recalls how phenomenological flesh produces sensory feedback even in the absence of direct touch. The *Cryobook Archives* thus reverse the domination and appropriation of flesh from the past and engenders a feeling of ethical

29 Patricia Louie and Rita Wilkes, "Representation of Race and Skin Tone in Medical Textbook Imagery," *Social Science & Medicine* 202 (2018): 39.

30 Ibid., 39.

relationality between the patient and viewers of her books. The blank pages of the books further invite viewers to remember the innumerable lost voices and stories behind the illustrations of anatomy. In its objectification, this flesh achieves a new kind of multiple subjectivity.

A Reunion of Art and Medicine

As evidenced by the exquisite images in anatomical treatises, artists were integral members of medical institutions for centuries. Their draftsmanship and ability to translate gross anatomy into the crisp lines of woodcut or engraving were essential skills to disseminate medical thought, while the deft inclusion of allegory and philosophy made these images meaningful and significant to their contemporary audiences (for better or for worse). Artists were fixtures within the anatomical theater and worked closely with physicians and anatomists to represent their work. However, as photography, medical imaging, and digital design illustration began to specialize, artists were edged out of medicine. The role of medically inclined artists then shifted from co-producers of medical education to visualizing illness experiences. Like Lyons and Duff, these artists take up the traditions of the past to shed new light on the medical paradigms that objectify patients in the present. In recent decades, however, space is being made to reintroduce arts methodologies back into medical education to hone the humanities facet of practicing medicine, promote empathy, and shift culture toward patient-centered care.

In an effort to move away from harmful biases and promote *reflexivity* within the institution of medicine, theologians, ethicists, and philosophers began promoting the inclusion of humanities alongside of clinical training in the 1960s.[31] Reflexivity involves continuously scrutinizing one's methods, positionality, and assumptions throughout practice and research in order to assess their ethics and efficacy. In such institutional introspections, the

31 Jane Macnaughton, "Medical Humanities Challenge to Medicine," *Journal of Evaluation in Medical Practice* 17, no. 5 (2011): 927–932.

arts and humanities are useful to promote the voices of patients, thereby contextualizing medicine within a much wider cultural makeup and societal impacts. To promote more holistic medical practices, these instructors focused on adding interdisciplinary studies back into medical education, more resembling the education of Renaissance anatomists than a singular focus of biomedical sciences. Such efforts, while admirable, were ultimately mired in challenges from the academic institution to justify the transfer of resources, time, and prove the efficacy of such curriculum changes.[32] The field of medical humanities has had difficulty finding widespread integration because of these debates ever since.[33]

Considering all of the ways artistic inquiry addresses some of the most systemic concerns in Western medicine, there remains a reluctance to fully integrate the humanities into healthcare education. This is because, although both art and medicine seek to elucidate the human condition, the methods of doing so rest within fundamentally different paradigms. Whereas medical science sits upon a legacy of uncovering truths about the natural world, art rests on the formulation of aesthetics that viewers find meaningful and significant to their worldview, which may then be questioned, reaffirmed, changed, or discarded. The subjectivity of the arts may be seen as problematic for a singular-truth, objectivity-seeking science, though it is precisely subjectivity that patients wish to foster with their physicians.

An example of such disparities is provided by bioethicist Jeffrey Bishop, who notes that the reticence to shift funds and resources to an integrated medical humanities education is because the discipline has yet to prove its effectiveness at improving medical practice in a longitudinal scientific study.[34] Such objective evidence may be impossible to gather for arts-based research, whose impacts on expanding students' worldview and promoting empathy may only tacitly reveal themselves over time and in immeasurable ways. Educational institutions demonstrate a bias toward quantifiable outcomes, which undermines the intrinsic and potentially transformative value

32 A closer look at these debates and difficulties with providing evidence-based justifications for the intrinsic value of art is provided in Chapter 4.

33 Macnaughton, "Medical Humanities Challenge to Medicine," 934.

34 Jeff Bishop, "Rejecting Medical Humanism: Medical Humanities and the Metaphysics of Medicine," *The Journal of Medical Humanities* 29 (2008): 23.

of the arts. If "every type of thinking must stand before the judgment seat of science,"[35] then the potentiality of the humanities to provoke reflexivity around Western medicine's divisive history and current hierarchical power structures will be forfeited.

Such an undervaluation of arts methodologies was encountered by UK artist and medical humanities instructor Christine Borland, who recounted in our interview that she "was quite personally offended by the attitude of some of the medical staff who would not hesitate to say to students in front of [her], 'Why are you wasting your time doing something like [art]? You are one of our best students, why are you doing something that you won't get any credit for?' "[36] A focus on utility, in this case, credit toward a medical degree, demonstrates a misconception for the intrinsic value of the arts and also discounts the role of arts experts like Borland, who understand not only how and why research-creation and interdisciplinary thinking ought to be integrated with medical learning, but also the history and philosophical reasoning behind such principles.

Medical students have also been shown to demonstrate bias against the humanities. Medical students may resist the pursuit of open questioning within medical humanities studies because they believe "medicine is an objective, scientific pursuit based almost exclusively on factual knowledge and technical skills."[37] Shapiro's survey of medical humanities students found that they complained of being forced into uncomfortable situations that confront their own vulnerabilities and fears. As well, "many refer to humanities teaching as pointless, boring, worthless, or just plain stupid."[38] Ultimately, "both anecdotal and investigational data suggest that medical humanities faculty have failed to adequately convince students that the medical humanities really matter to them as future physicians."[39] Clearly, more investment in how medical humanities is taught, who teaches it,

35 Ibid., 17.

36 Christine Borland, interview by Darian Goldin Stahl, February 19, 2019.

37 Johanna Shapiro, "Medical Humanities and Their Discontents: Definitions, Critiques, and Implications," *Academic Medicine* 84, no. 2 (2009): 193.

38 Ibid., 192.

39 Ibid., 193.

methods of engagement, and clarity on its rationale is necessary to demonstrate the intrinsic value of humanities and arts in medicine.

Proposing a methodology for interdisciplinary teams to generate research results and pedagogies via artistic outputs, the authors of *Parallaxic Practice*[40] provide valuable rationales for approaching the same healthcare topic from distinct disciplinary backgrounds. Parallaxic praxis involves collaborating researchers analyzing the same set of creative or subjective data, often generated by community members with lived experience of the topic, using their various expertises and coming to shared understanding of its significance to the research question. This research design strategy treats artistic outputs as potential healthcare data, rather than simply a therapeutic practice for makers. Like an in-depth review of artists' books to examine systemic biases in medical culture, "integrating the arts in research methodology affords scholars new lenses for viewing, analyzing, representing, and disseminating research."[41] Significant and meaningful, parallaxic praxis thus elevates the status of art as worthy of investigation for improving healthcare policies or studying the effects of illness and disability. Honoring methodological pluralism breaks down the "us versus them" mentality that tends to mire health humanities research and fosters a sense of co-learning between art, medicine, and community.

Co-teaching courses with art and medical experts is way to exemplify parallaxic practice. For example, Brown University medical students were offered a co-taught cross-listed course with Rhode Island School of Design students. Collaborating with art students and engaging with the field's methods like regular formative group critiques, the students practiced openly questioning their own methods and decisions. The medical professor for this course, Jay Baruch, observed that making art encouraged students to scrutinize their discomfort, to "make mistakes, to embrace failure as a valuable and utterly integral part of the learning process."[42] Another example comes to us from Bournemouth University, where a photography course was offered to general practitioner trainees. Attempting

40 Sameshima, Maarhuis, and Wiebe, *Parallaxic Practice.*

41 Ibid., 2.

42 Jay Baruch and Kelli Auerbach, "Beyond Comfort Zones: An Experiment in Medical and Art Education," *Journal for Learning Through the Arts* 8, no. 1 (2012): 9.

to capture the effects of medical practices on film was found to reveal and productively engage with the high emotions of their profession. Co-professor Rutherford's expertise in photography enabled him to overcome the trainees' initial "degree of hesitation or reticence" for this "touchy feely stuff."[43] In our interview, he attests, "without somebody who was confidently and knowledgeably and emotionally open to lead them through the process, I don't think it would have worked."[44] In both cases, the artists' expertise in navigating research-creation in conjunction with experts in medical sciences was critical to promote the buy-in necessary to initiate reflexivity.[45] Taking seriously the notion that artistic methods can instigate valuable research has the potential to influence a culture of medicine that values the suppression of emotion in favor of more open engagements with the human side of healthcare practices.

One final example of parallaxic practice is provided by the artist Laura Ferguson and her return to the anatomical theater as New York University School of Medicine's long-term artist in residence. Ferguson leads weekly anatomy drawing classes of the cadavers the students dissect during their medical degrees. Practically, she concludes that the close looking involved in drawing from life fosters the students' ability to more accurately recognize the subtle structures of anatomy. Intrinsically, the meditative, durational time of drawing also gives students space to process the brutal and emotionally laden act of dissection, which may otherwise negatively impact mental health.[46] The extracurricular time and care it takes to accurately draw anatomical structures "is part of a growing movement in medicine that encourages a more empathetic attitude towards patients and recognizes the value of listening to their voices, especially through the expressive power of arts."[47] Spending time creating art that honors the patient, as we will see

43 Rutherford, interview by Darian Goldin Stahl, February 5, 2019.

44 Ibid.

45 Rutherford, et al., "Using Photography to Enhance GP Trainees' Reflective Practice and Professional Development," *Journal of Medical Humanities* 44, no. 3 (2018): 158–164.

46 Laura Ferguson and Katie Grogan, *Art & Anatomy: Drawings* (San Francisco: University of California Medical Humanities Press, 2017), 15.

47 Ibid., 12.

in subsequent chapters on artists' books in the medical classroom, has the power to reverse dehumanizing detachment, acknowledge the emotions of medicine, and create space to be in relation with their patients.

While co-teaching or artist-led initiatives demonstrate the meaning-making value of distinct disciplinary experts circling the same healthcare topic, this model of pedagogy can be fraught with imbalances of workload and compensation. Professor of Medical Humanities Alan Bleakley points out that "the older 'medical humanities' for too long have lived off the good will of artists and designers who would provide their labor, intelligence and creative flair for the benefit of medicine or medical education without the medical community giving something back to the arts and design communities."[48] Science and Technology Studies Professor Charlotte Sleigh also warns of the hierarchies at play within art and medical/science collaborations, which are influenced by, in addition to the above, what are considered "legitimate" research methods and unequal time investments.[49] The push for collaboration without addressing such imbalanced partnerships, as critical medical humanities author Patricia Waugh cautions, "may insidiously preserve the knowledge hierarchies of the positivist legacy"[50] in medicine, and ultimately only reinforce disciplinary divisions. If humanities and arts experts are not invited to become full and balanced collaborative partners in these pedagogies, then medical humanities curricula risk becoming superficial adaptations of artistic methods—a balm or "helpful friend" to the stresses of medical education—and ultimately undermine the potentiality of medical humanities to guide the hearts and minds of new generations of physicians.

48 Alan Bleakley, "Transitions in Health Humanities: Towards a 'Critical' Health Humanities that Embraces Beauty," in *Insight 2: Engaging the Health Humanities*, eds. Lianne McTavish and Pamela Brett-McLean (Edmonton: University of Alberta Department of Art and Design, 2013), 12.

49 Charlotte Sleigh and Sarah Craske, "Nine-Tenths of the Iceberg: Research as the Unseen Component of Artists' Work," *Interalia Magazine* (November 2017): 1.

50 Patricia Waugh, "Afterward: Evidence and Experiment," in *The Edinburgh Companion to the Critical Medical Humanities*, eds. Anne Whitehead and Angela Woods (Edinburgh: Edinburgh University, 2018).

Conclusion

Those who possess books, and to a much greater extent, those who make books, hold the power of knowledge representation. In the long arc of medical books and illustration, members of elite institutions have defined what being ill or well looks like until very recently. Artists' books challenge the institution to recognize that the historical visual cultures of medicine "were little more than tools used to justify the domination of white European (and American) males over colonized populations, women, and People of Color," which have resulted in lingering biases to this day.[51] A strategy to alert readers to the overt and subtle biases engrained within biomedical images is to continuously critique their origins and methods of influence. The artist's goal in appropriating images and practices of bygone medicine is to take the power of bodily representation, and then alter, transform, and return it with renewed attention to the lived, sensing body.

I have situated the longitudinal perspective of medical books against contemporary artists' books from Lyons and Duff to show how, although enormous advances have been made toward health equity in recent decades, the foundational power structures of Western medicine continue to hold uneven sway over the lives of patients today. Gendered biases rooted in the Renaissance still put undue pressure on women patients amidst medical paternalism. The representations of skin color in medical textbooks continue to demonstrate a white bias, and do not reflect the racial distribution of modern society. Finally, the objectification of bodies neglects the patient's voice and sense of agency, particularly after death. Such enduring biases lead artists to take up the images and practices of the past in an effort to insert a critical and authoritative voice into the politics of health. In addition to fostering a sense of community with others who have felt similar pressures navigating our healthcare system, generative arts methodologies are beginning to be incorporated within medical institutions. Taking the

51 Thomas Cole, Nathan Carlin, and Ronald Carson, *Medical Humanities: An Introduction* (Cambridge: Cambridge University Press, 2014), 5.

form of reflexive pedagogies, these innovative collaborations do shy away from the challenges presented by artists.

Advocating for partnerships between the arts and medicine shifts artists from critical outsiders to integral co-researchers. Collaborating perspectives within a parallaxic practice allow for ambiguity and open-ended questioning of how health knowledge is culturally constructed and upheld. By analyzing medical images, reading patient narrative, studying artworks, *making* artwork, and many other forms of humanities interventions, remerging art and medicine is a strategy of turning the dominating medical gaze onto itself. In critical arts practices, learners may become more reflexive toward the power structures and paradigms of medicine and practice more holistic care for patients and themselves.

CHAPTER 4

Research-Creation in Patients' Artists' Books

Introduction: *Field Notes: How to Be With*

Field Notes: How to Be With is the artist's book I created during my investigation of art and health. This chapter is framed through a close phenomenological reading of this artist's book to demonstrate how research-creation can be implemented as a generative methodology. I also exemplify how artists' books are particularly well suited for capturing sensory and experiential investigations. *Field Notes* structures expert interviews, archive research, and artistic collaborations within the paginated format to explore critical health humanities practices today.

Research-creation is a geographically Canadian, and Montreal-based in particular, term for the kinds of evidence and knowing that can only occur through artistic processes.[1] Other names and articulations for this methodology in North America and the UK include arts-based research, arts-led research, artistic inquiry, a/r/tography, among many others.[2] A common thread throughout these terms is that open, abstract questions in combination with a methodological approach to art making are found to result in a high potential for interdisciplinary innovation and creative problem solving.

Although creating art has always been a methodology for investigating the given world, experience, or cognition, it is only recently (the 1990s in Canada) that creating art as a method and output of research was formally recognized by universities in the form of a PhD, as well as new streams of research funding

1 Natalie Loveless, *How to Make Art at the End of the World: A Manifesto for Research-Creation* (Durham: Duke University Press, 2019), 4.

2 Patricia Leavy, *Method Meets Art: Arts-Based Research Practice* (New York City: Guilford Press, 2015), 5.

from federal organizations like the Social Sciences and Humanities Research Council (SSHRC). US proponents like Patricia Leavy,[3] Shaun McNiff,[4] Eliot Eisner,[5] and Susan Finley[6] continue to form conceptual rationales and pragmatic methods for conducting arts-based research. Canadian scholars like Natalie Loveless,[7] Erin Manning,[8] Kim Sawchuk, and Owen Chapman[9] nuance and analyze the potentiality of research-creation to form new knowledge. As well, medical humanities collaborators Jane Macnaughton and Havi Carel[10] capitalize on the exhibition of research-creation outcomes as public health outreach regarding stigmatized health conditions.

The research-creation conducted for *Field Notes* brings together two embedded fieldwork contexts: first as a Visiting Scholar in the University of Kent Medical Humanities Program in Canterbury, England, and then as the Artist in Residence at the McGill University Fertility Research Laboratory in Montreal, Canada. I was drawn to conduct a portion of my fieldwork in the UK because of what I perceive to be the highly developed level of scholarship addressing arts-based research in healthcare. I was also most interested in collaborating with Dr. Stella Bolaki, who is the Director of the University of Kent's Medical Humanities Program and has published chapters

3 Ibid.
4 Shaun McNiff, "Art-Based Research," in *Handbook of the Arts in Qualitative Research: Perspectives, Methodologies, Examples, and Issues*, eds. J. Gary Knowles and Ardra L. Cole (Los Angeles: Sage Publications, 2008), 29–40.
5 Elliot W. Eisner, "On the Differences between Scientific and Artistic Approaches to Qualitative Research," *Review of Research in Visual Arts Education* 7, no. 1 (1981): 7.
6 Susan Finley, "Arts-Based Research," in *Handbook of the Arts in Qualitative Research: Perspectives, Methodologies, Examples, and Issues*, eds. J Gary Knowles and Ardra L. Cole (Los Angeles: Sage Publications, 2008), 71–82.
7 Loveless, *How to Make Art at the End of the World.*
8 Erin Manning, "Ten Propositions for Research-Creation," in *Collaboration in Performance Practice*, eds. Noyale Colin and Stefanie Sachsenmaier (London: Palgrave Macmillan, 2016), 133–141.
9 Owen Chapman and Kim Sawchuk, "Research-Creation: Intervention, Analysis and 'Family Resemblances,'" *Canadian Journal of Communication* 37 (2012): 1–22.
10 Jane Macnaughton and Havi Carel, "Breathing and Breathlessness in Clinic and Culture: Using Critical Medical Humanities to Bridge an Epistemic Gap," in *The Edinburgh Companion to the Medical Humanities*, eds. Anne Whitehead and Angela Woods (Edinburgh: Edinburgh University Press, 2016), 294–309.

and numerous articles on the potentiality of artists' books in healthcare research. As a Visiting Scholar, I was also able to study the University of Kent's Prescriptions Collection: a distinctive archive of artists' books dedicated to topics of bodily concern. These books enabled me to investigate the multiplicity of methods artists employ to communicate their encounters with medicine, as well as how these books are employed as primary health research material in university coursework. Throughout this chapter, I will position the artists' books from this collection that I found to be especially poignant for my arguments on the communicative aspects of bookness and phenomenology, and which ultimately influenced the final formation of *Field Notes*.

While in the UK, I took this geographical opportunity to meet and formally interview over twenty scholars working at the nexus of humanities and health, including artists, writers, physicians, historians, librarians, and philosophers. My goal with these interviews was to discover the most emergent themes and arguments in contemporary health humanities, as well as if and how research-creation is being employed as a research methodology. Portions of these interviews have been transcribed and rearranged in *Field Notes* as if these researchers were sharing in a discourse with one another. The interweaving of these voices portrays the interconnectedness of thought on these topics.

In my other research position as Artist in Residence at the McGill University Fertility Research Laboratory, I shadowed two scientists for three months, observed their daily experiments, attended their progress report meetings, and held numerous informal conversations with them about their research. My first aim in this residency was to better understand the process of generating original medical knowledge, and how the scientists' sensing bodies are implicated in, or are displaced from, embodied perception. My second objective for this residency was to use aesthetics as a meeting point between science and arts-based research: to bridge the lacuna between the images produced in a laboratory and how the end users of medicine (i.e., patients) re-present their own imaged bodies in artists' books. Many of the images included in *Field Notes* emerged from a collaborative printmaking process I developed with these two scientists.

Field Notes exemplifies the benefits of research-creation methodologies. Although it is accompanied by this written chapter, I consider *Field Notes* to be equally rigorous and potentially more eminent due to its compact format and intimate impact, which may be more capable of speaking to a wider range of audiences than this written component. It is in part a thesis that weaves together facets of arguments from preeminent scholars of the field. It is also a collaborative ethnographic piece of fine art. It is research about art-based research. It could therefore best be described as research-creation on the process and outcomes of research-creation—an embodied analysis of how artists' books embody ideas. This is different than the largely auto-ethnographic research-creation that occurs in most artists' books about illness, where makers seek to materialize and communicate an inscrutable phenomenon about themselves, as is the general aim of the books I encountered in the Prescriptions Collection. Although these books are also textual and multi-sensory investigations of illness, *Field Notes* goes a step further to embed artists' books within a wider discourse about the state of arts-based research in healthcare, who employs it, and who would benefit from doing so. It is a meta-book on the process and outcomes of making books.

The purpose of *Field Notes* alongside this accompanying chapter is to argue for research-creation artists' books as original critical health humanities scholarship. The unique contribution of artists' books to the field is their ability to express lived experience and foster intercorporealities with the reader through the intertwining of materiality, text, and image. The neglect of this kind of embodied scholarship within healthcare is of growing concern, as biomedical imaging and other technologically mediated ways of examining the body contribute to a sense of depersonalization from both patients and healthcare providers.[11] The multivalent modalities of artists' books challenge healthcare researchers to de-center linguistic narrative and third-person case studies as the modus operandi of illness research, and "forge new alliances with the arts and humanities in order to remain pluralistic and experimental."[12] Returning attention to the sensorium enables a phenomenological practice of understanding illness, empathy, and creative care.

11 Drew Leder, *The Distressed Body: Rethinking Illness, Imprisonment, and Healing* (Chicago: The University of Chicago Press, 2016), 44.

12 Stella Bolaki, *Illness as Many Narratives: Arts, Medicine, and Culture* (Edinburgh: Edinburgh University Press, 2016), 7.

Given the transcendental nature of books, that is, the medium's long history in our society that has cultivated certain norms and expectations of what a book is and does, closely analyzing artists' books concludes with the impossibility of reading them in isolation. Artists' books depend on a culturally engrained knowledge of how to read a book in order to turn such standards on their head. Subverting our preconceived notions for bookness is a core method for artists to illuminate lived experiences that counter our preconceived notions of health and illness. Therefore, the artists' books cited here portray entangled perspectives that are at once far reaching and intensely personal, variable, and dependent upon a multitude of potential interpretations from each successive reader. To create a potential meaning that illuminates some aspect of the artists' experiences, I employ a phenomenological practice of sensory description and material hermeneutics. While acknowledging the subjectivity of the medium, artists' books are an *experience*, of which this is mine.

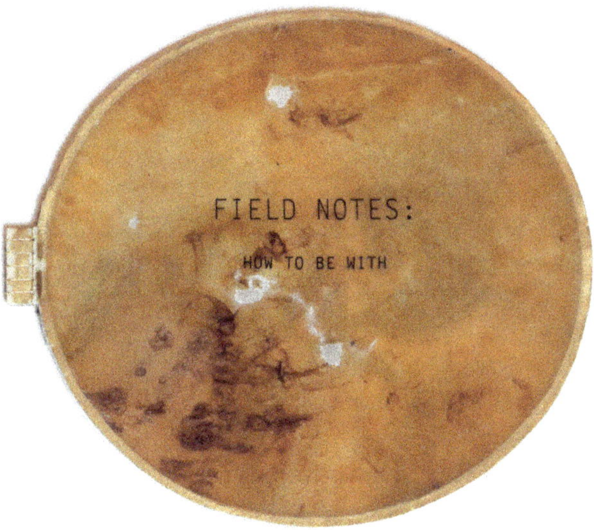

Figure 4.1: Darian Goldin Stahl, *Field Notes: How to Be With*, Toner transfer on waxed silk, 8″ × 8″, 2020.

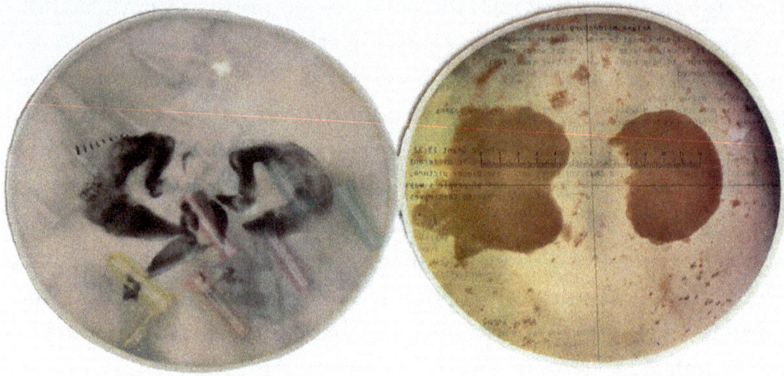

Figure 4.2: Darian Goldin Stahl, *Field Notes: How to Be With*, 2020.

Sensory Meaning-Making in Artists' Books

When closed, *Field Notes: How to Be With* is an 8-inch round book and about one-fourth of an inch thick. Across the center one can read the title, *Field Notes: How to Be With*, in an unadorned sans serif font (see Figure 4.1). Around the outer edge of the cover is a golden ring. The book is bound on the left-hand side with golden thread in a Japanese or stab-stitch binding. Beneath the binding one can see a golden stencil of the metal hardware that tightens an embroidery hoop. This detail gives some context for the unusual shape, though its inclusion is unobtrusive enough to evoke many other interpretations for the round cover.

The book's shape is immediately arresting because it differs from the typical rectangular book form. Its roundness is not geometrically perfect and therefore feels more natural in origin, like a planetary body or cross section of a tree. The cover shifts hues between warm ochres and umbers—reminiscent of deer leather. In some places, especially on the back cover of the book, there is a topography of shallow bumps, bubbles, and crags. These features make the leathery cover appear burned or afflicted with some kind of skin condition. Overall, the cover is easily understood as the skin of book-body—be it human or nonhuman in origin.

The multiple interpretations of this cover initiate the idea that all objects belong within networks of meanings, associations, and histories, the circle being perhaps the most fundamental shape in human consciousness. This assertion is based on Barbara Maria Stratford's book, *Echo Objects* (2007), which argues that the human brain solicits common shapes and patterns in order to make sense of the world. What could be a more recognizable shape than the round eye of a loved one or gazing upon the moon? In fine art, the simplest geometric forms, like the circle, are often the most meaning-full compositions because we have called upon its geometry over and over again. As Stafford attests, "this graphic grammar, composed of discrete character or cipher combinations, allows us to generate a range of denotative and connotative meanings from elementary forms."[13] More specifically for the topics of this book, the circle connotes the scientific composition of the body (parts) seen through the microscope, fluoroscopy scan, or surgical cameras. This, along with the potentially pathological-looking skin of the cover, alerts us to medical themes to come.

Opening the front cover, the book becomes a diptych (see Figure 4.2). Splitting the circular book and forming a binocular view of the book-body alludes to all the partnerships that have informed this research: art and science, myself and my sister, objects and subjects, health and illness. The ways in which all of these seemingly dualistic topics are actually intimately intertwined, constitutive and informing of one another, becomes clear through the embodied gesture of lifting each translucent page to placing it upon its opposite.

13 Barbara Maria Stafford, *Echo Objects: The Cognitive Work of Images* (Chicago: The University of Chicago Press, 2007), 20.

The first section of the pages contains two small figures curled toward each other in the fetal position. Only the very surface of figures' torsos is shown, which gives the impression of a planar slice from an MRI or CT scan. The appearance of spines and other anatomy furthers the associations with biomedical imaging technologies. These two figures are nestled within two larger kidney bean shapes. Flipping the page, the figures are lifted away to join the multi-colored testing vials on the left side of the diptych. The presence of crosshairs and a measuring guide across the shapes clue us in that they may be very small organs viewed through a microscope. They are in fact mouse ovaries.

This visual introduction of *Field Notes* exhibits the two major visual collaborations that occurred in the making of this book: between myself and my sister, and between myself and two fertility scientists at McGill University. *Field Notes* is the latest iteration of my long-term collaborative art practice with my sister, Devan Stahl, who is a hospital chaplain, Professor of Medical Ethics at Baylor University, a chronically ill person with multiple sclerosis, and was struggling with infertility during the course of this research. I began making artwork about Devan's symptoms of MS and sharing them with her in 2012 because I found the topic of disease and all the implications it had for my sister's life too difficult to acknowledge directly. By creating these works and gifting them to her, I was able to *show* her my care in a way that my words had failed. This artistic gesture inspired Devan to write more narratives about her lived experiences of illness and procure copies of her MRI scans to share with me. She thought we could creatively expand these singular-purpose images to also communicate the impacts of illness on her daily life. Through the layering and additive processes of printmaking and bookmaking, I merge her MRI scans with impressions of my own skin in an attempt to provide shelter to her imaged viscera. This blending of our bodies is the two figures that appear in the beginning of *Field Notes*, and they embody the creative caretaking I share with my sister.

After years of semi-annual MRI scans and demanding clinical trials, Devan's experiences under medical surveillance compounded during her years-long effort to become a mother. She had to discontinue her

MS medications, as their potential effects on a fetus are unknown. This put her health in a state of constant precarity, and she felt an incredible amount of pressure to become pregnant quickly—which did not happen. My care for Devan continued to include reimaginings of her medicalized body, which now incorporated time-lapsed fluoroscopy stills of contrast being injected into her uterus, and eventually, the first ultrasounds of her son.

Representing the complexity of illness is one of the main goals of this research-creation, and although there is no research that links MS with infertility, it would be wrong to say they are unrelated. Forgoing vital medications for years in the hopes of conceiving a child is not an easy choice to make, and these decisions were also interrogated by her physicians, particularly in light of her "advanced maternal age." The inclusion of Devan's medical scans exemplifies for the readers the pressures patients face, particularly for women, to lead the life of their choosing while also being ill.

The mouse ovaries and various assemblages of medical ephemera printed throughout the book are the result of my second fine art collaboration with two scientists at the McGill University Fertility Research Laboratory, Karen Carvalho and Sofia Granados. Acknowledging my lack of knowledge about such topics, I sought out this residency in order to understand current and future fertility treatment possibilities that may go on to help people like my sister. I was also curious about the people constructing primary scientific knowledge, as this perspective was generally absent from my health humanities research thus far. My research questions at the center of this artist residency ask, "What is at stake when the images of medical and scientific research contain so much specialized knowledge that they become indecipherable by the people they are meant to help? How can these images be deconstructed and contextualized in ways that shed light on lived experience?" And finally, "How might aesthetics form a bridge between scientists and those who seek healing?"

To engage these questions, I performed what design anthropologist Sarah Pink defines as "sensory ethnography," which is "an emplaced ethnography that attends to the questions of experience by accounting for the relationships between bodies, minds, and the materiality and sensoriality of the environment."[14] To know a place, it is best to experience it through prolonged presence, touch, smell, and sound. To know the practices of a person who operates within that particular space, such as this laboratory, ideally the researcher performs the practice alongside the practitioner's expertise. In this position alongside, each person contributes her own situated knowledge into a potentially collaborative environment.

My sustained presence in the lab established trust and rapport with the scientists. I could ask probing questions about the process and implications of their research in the midst of its occurrence—creating a far richer sensory understanding than typical sit-down interviews. I asked questions like, "What is this experiment hoping to discover? How does it feel to conduct research using the ova of mice versus the ova of humans? How might what you are doing today impact patients in the future? What is your experience as a woman in science? What are the future plans for this research, and for yourself?"

What I had not anticipated were the emotional stakes of conducting scientific research. My own preconceived notions of hushed, antiseptic environments and stoic objectivity were completely upended. When real people donate their harvested ova or mice have been specially bred and sacrificed for dissection, the pressure to successfully carry out experiments is incredibly high. I also learned that, in spite of its advanced robotic or technological portrayals in popular media, much of the procedure for scientific experiments is conducted through carefully orchestrated body movements. I observed, most notably, how they pulled their breath through a rubber tube connected to a handcrafted glass pipette (which they fired and pulled themselves) in order to carefully lift a single mouse ovum from a Petri dish and place it into the experiment's chemicals, all while only viewing this minute action through a microscope. Finally, it became abundantly evident the depth of creativity needed to even begin formulating an experiment, how to conduct it using incontestable scientific methods, and then accurately imaging and interpreting its results in order to inform the next day's experiment. By the end of my residency, I found the laboratory

14 Sarah Pink, *Doing Sensory Ethnography* (Los Angeles: Sage Publishing Ltd., 2015), 28.

to be a space where sensory engagement and creativity thrive, which makes sustained art/sci collaborations all the more possible.

To form a true collaboration rather than a one-way transmission of knowledge, I invited the scientists into my art studio to discover how aesthetics might join our disciplines, and potentially, form new knowledges at a nexus of art and science. We first gathered the daily tools of their research, like colorful syringes, nitrile gloves, and biohazard bags, to create aesthetic assemblages on the photo bed of a scanner. I then taught them my encaustic printmaking technique, which allowed us to layer and merge our Xerox scans with other appropriated images from the history of medicine or the scientists' own microscopy. Although I was not permitted to photograph the mice in the laboratory, I stitched their visages with golden thread into the prints as a way to pay homage to their lives in this research-creation.

The method of collaging these images together, as art education professor Kathleen Vaughan states, "with its overlappings, juxtapositions, and shifting centers and margins—can be seen as a transborder practice with epistemological implications."[15] For example, the scientists' motivation for collaboration was to connect what they do in the laboratory with the communities they serve, and demystify the scientific process for a general audience. Especially in this current political climate of science skepticism or denial, making science scrutable to non-experts is an essential strategy to convey the importance of their research. I argue that including the images and practices of science in an artist's book, which invites the viewer to activate and become a part of its meaning, is a productive way to form inclusive alliances with the public. The translucent pages within this artist's book can be seen as participatory collages, as the reader activates the layers of image and text by viewing through them, pulling them apart, reading them individually, and placing them back into their seat. Ultimately, the narrow and big-picture applications of the scientists' findings are made more apparent through the layered and collaged pages of *Field Notes*. This method of meaning-making implicates both artistic and scientific epistemologies,

15 Kathleen Vaughan, "Pieced Together: Collage as an Artist's Method for Interdisciplinary Research," *International Journal of Qualitative Methods* 4 (2005): 32.

and portrays the mass amount of labor, materials, and creativity necessary to produce the images of our shared research.

From the beginning of this residency, my goal was to understand how the narrow results of an experiment link within networks of discoveries that finally go on to impact people like my sister, the real-world receivers of treatment. In short, capturing the bigger picture. Collaging and binding the images of science into an artist's book destabilizes and abstracts their original, narrow context so that new associations can emerge. The movement of transparent bodies across the spine of the book keeps the images suspended, and the ambiguities of scale and origins of body parts sustain such instabilities. The corporeal fluidity of *Field Notes* disrupts the boundaries between human and nonhuman and layers them back onto the other as mutually constitutive. This pagination connects the restricted space of the laboratory with the impacts of scientific research on patients, families, and the researchers themselves. This is how *Field Notes* is able to bridge the epistemological divides of art and science, and how it will continue to engage current and future practices in health humanities.

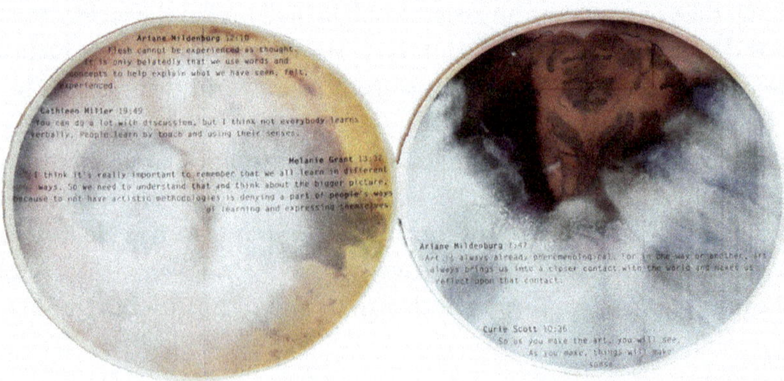

Figure 4.3: Darian Goldin Stahl, *Field Notes: How to Be With*, 2020.

Ariane Mildenburg 12:10

Flesh cannot be experienced as thought. It is only belatedly that we use words and concepts to help explain what we have seen, felt, experienced.

Cathleen Miller 19:49

You can do a lot with discussion, but I think not everybody learns verbally. People learn by touch and using their senses.

Melanie Grant 13:32

I think it's really important to remember that we all learn in different ways. So we need to understand that and think about the bigger picture, because to not have artistic methodologies is denying a part of people's ways of learning and expressing themselves.

Ariane Mildenburg 7:47

Art is always already phenomenological. For in one way or another, art always brings us into a closer contact with the world and makes us reflect upon that contact.

Curie Scott 10:36

So as you make the art, you will *see*. As you *make,* things will make sense.

Figure 4.3 depicts the first text included in *Field Notes*. The speaker's name is printed along with the timestamp from our recording. I aligned the segments of text along opposite sides of the page to evoke stereo sound within the reader's head as the voices bounce back and forth, which I have also reprinted above in a similar fashion. This spread alerts the reader to the sensory aspects of this artist's book and how they are implicated in learning.

The materials of *Field Notes* are meant to provide meaning in excess of the book's imagery and text. As Classen points out, "many feelings are difficult to put into language, they are too subtle or too powerful or too complex. The anthropology of the senses sensitizes us to the mutable ways in which humans communicate and express themselves through nonlinguistic modalities."[16] The value of this kind of expression is to challenge normative

16 Constance Classen, *The Deepest Sense: A Cultural History of Touch* (Chicago: University of Illinois Press, 2012), xvii.

styles of scholarship, like written theses, which can be inaccessible and unintelligible to non-specialist audiences. An academic reliance on text neglects sensory ways of knowing—a gap that artists' books are exceptionally suited to fill.

Apart from the visual and haptic description provided above, a reader may first notice that *Field Notes* feels heavier than anticipated. This is due to the saturation of wax imbued within each page that transforms the underlying silk substrate into a translucent cross section of flesh. While wax has long been used to imitate the pallor and translucency of flesh in anatomical modeling, another significant sensory contribution of the wax is its exhalation of aroma. The darker material of the covers also contains dissolved sugars, a sweet caramel scent that is further nuanced by a covering of beeswax. In addition to this scent, many of the internal pages of *Field Notes* are covered in a wax medium that uses turpentine as its mineral spirit, whose remarkable pine perfume remains embedded in the wax long after the spirit has evaporated. The touch and smell of this book remind the reader of its materiality by surprising the senses at every turn.

Scent is a method to literally enter the interiority of the reader and connect with their emotions. Verbeek and Campen explain that "more than any other sense, smell can instantly determine an atmosphere or a mood, almost independent of the context."[17] The pleasant scents of *Field Notes* have the potential to provide sensory care for the reader during what may otherwise be an uneasy read on illness. Care for the body through sweet scents is an ancient idea, as the dominant pre-modern concept for how diseased traveled was through *miasma*, or vaporized matter that carried disease via stench. Therefore, a strategy for staving off disease was to overpower it with other pungent or pleasant aromas.[18] During instances of plague in London, Classen relays that "amid the strength of disease and death, lavender, juniper and cinnamon were burnt in the streets and houses to 'cleanse' the air of infection."[19] The fragrances of *Field Notes,* in addition

17 Caro Verbeek and Cretien van Campen, "Inhaling Memories: Smell and Taste Memories in Art, Science, and Practice," *Senses and Society* 8, no. 2 (2013): 137.

18 Steven Connor, *The Book of Skin* (London: Reaction Books Ltd., 2004), 213.

19 Constance Classen, *The Museum of the Senses* (London: Bloomsbury Academic, 2017), 112.

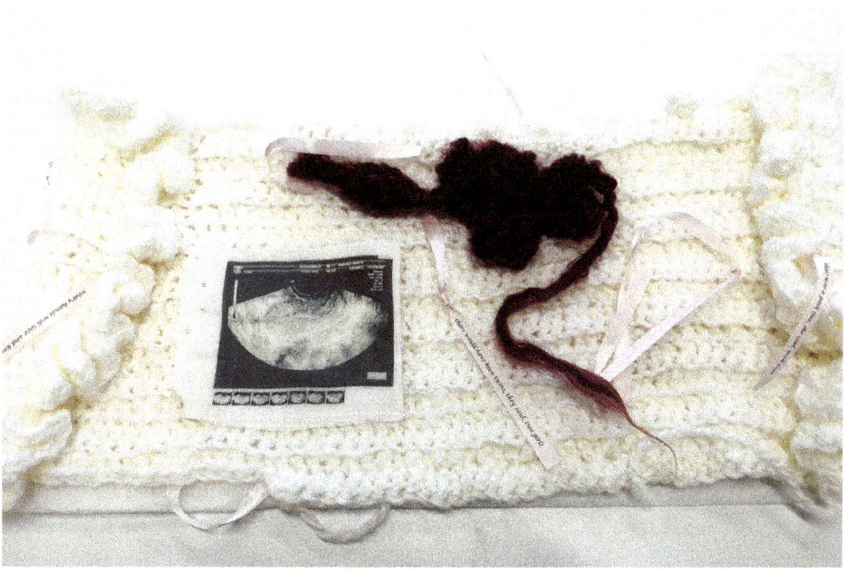

Figure 4.4: Erin K. Schmidt, *The Unfinished Blanket*, Crocheted cotton yarn, inkjet-printed ribbon, inkjet-printed silk, 10″ × 7.5″ × 3″, 2016.

to the anatomical associations of wax modeling, are a method to intertwine such past and present conceptualizations of medicine.

Strong scents elicit some of our deepest memories, a phenomenon that occurs "largely independent of personal will, breaking into the conscious mind unbidden and at unexpected moments."[20] What does the aroma of caramel evoke for you? What emotions rise to the surface when surrounded by the scent of pine? Memories provoked by scent are typically tied to some of our oldest impressions, are often non-lingual, and may induce stronger emotions than viewing images alone.[21] Scent is a strategy to make present and personal all the various meanings and interpretations of this artist's book based upon each reader's history. At the very least, the scent of this book ensures a reader cannot engage with it and remain unaffected.

20 Verbeek and Campen, "Inhaling Memories," 135.
21 Ibid., 140.

Many of the over seventy artists' books within the Prescriptions Collection engage multiple senses as a strategy to tacitly communicate deeply emotional topics that are difficult to put into words, and perhaps none more so than Erin K. Schmidt's *The Unfinished Blanket* (see Figure 4.4). It is a white, fuzzy, delicately crocheted book comprised of a single "sheet" folded into thirds. It is so soft and light that it almost feels like I am touching nothing but air. Perhaps this lack of solid touch is my first entry point into this book on loss. Opening the covers, we first see a clumped strip of crimson yarn, then a scattering of fastened pink text-printed ribbons, and finally, a much smaller silk book sewn inside. This second internal book is printed with sonograms and text; however, I do not need to read the text to already comprehend that this book concerns the grieving of a miscarriage.

According to Schmidt's artist statement, the book pertains to "the joy and excitement of a new pregnancy, followed by the worry of a possible complication, and finally the deep sadness at the loss of not just one baby, but of twins due to a molar pregnancy."[22] Inside the smaller second book, phrases like "Three Copies of Chromosome 18//Antenatal loss//Rare"[23] are printed boundlessly around the page. Schmidt explains that "the words don't seem to make sense, but float on the page much the same way that confusing medical terminology and jargon seem to hang in the air without meaning when speaking with doctors during times of distress."[24] The ineffectual words from her physicians are visually communicated through their unmoored composition.

The extreme privacy of a miscarriage in our culture makes this relatively common occurrence nevertheless unutterable and even taboo to mourn publicly. It is no wonder, then, that Schmidt chooses to circumvent a cohesive narrative in favor of poetic and sensory meaning-making methods.

22 Erin Schmidt, "The Unfinished Blanket," accessed June 12, 2020, <https://www.erinkschmidt.com/theunfinishedblanket.html>.

23 Erin Schmidt, *The Unfinished Blanket*, Prescriptions Collection, University of Kent, Canterbury, 2016.

24 Schmidt, "The Unfinished Blanket."

Holding the unoccupied blanket in one's hands places the reader in a close relation with Schmidt, as the sadness of the event is made tangible. The handcrafted quality of the textile page shows the labor that went into the object for babies that would never experience it. However, the soft touch of the book might bring the reader (and hopefully, Schmidt herself) a bit of comfort amidst its mourning.

One of the most significant impacts of artists' books in healthcare research is their embodied share-ability, which overcomes the silence around topics like infertility and miscarriage. In a materialized form, the emotions of grief can be tacitly felt, held, and dispersed over a community of readers who may be similarly impacted with struggles to build a family or those comprehending the emotional impact of such an event on others for the first time. Drew Leder also attests to the healing qualities of handmade objects shared with others. "Such objects thus embody not only divine love but that of the community [...]. Here the touch of the shawl or quilt re-presents—makes present, over and over—a communal embrace."[25] Unlike machine-produced books, there is a tangible sense of the hands that craft the page for *The Unfinished Blanket*. It is as if we are able to touch and be touched by the maker over vast distances simply by holding their creation. This engagement of touch encourages a phenomenological intercorporeality that fosters empathy. Leder agrees that "unlike other sensory modes, touch unfolds through an impactful reciprocity between the toucher and the touched. For the ill person this can serve to establish human connection and assist therapeutic chance at the prelinguistic level."[26] The intercorporeality of haptic books like *The Unfinished Blanket* demonstrate the effectiveness of nonlinguistic research-creation to form intimate, emotive communication between subjects.

25 Leder, *The Distressed Body*, 76.
26 Ibid., 9.

Text in Artists' Books

Jane Macnaughton 18:32

So during the course of clinical interactions it is very important to be able to *see* the patient—to be interacting with the patient as a person. But it's also important as a professional clinician to be able to view the person objectively, as a thing that you're examining, as a piece of flesh you're trying to understand.

Rutherford 9:37

One of the issues that we found, and I'm sure that it was not unique to this particular group, is that many of the G.P.'s took refuge behind facades of objectivity and distance. It's obviously an issue. It's been well documented as a source of concern on the part of the patients that, "The doctors don't seem to care about me as a person. They see me as a complex of symptoms."

Veronique Chance 20:30

You realize how vulnerable you are when you're in that situation. You don't have the knowledge, you're being told, and you have to trust their judgment. You feel quite powerless.

Maria Vaccarella 8:51

The super accurate language, and you know, using all these kinds of rhetorical terms, we actually build a barrier rather than a bridge.

Rutherford 8:00

That barrier is often erected, consciously or unconsciously, would you prefer consciously or subconsciously, for the emotional protection of the G.P.

Melanie Grant 15:51

It's probably showing that they're not receiving the kind of holistic care that they need, as well as the practitioners who are dealing with the difficult situations all of the time.

The text in *Field Notes* serves to explicitly address the most emergent debates in the health humanities. A common topic throughout my interviews concerned the perceived damage or benefits of objectifying patients during the course of a clinical interaction. While this sense of being seen as a "piece of flesh" can be detrimental to patient satisfaction, critical medical humanities professor and MD Jane Macnaughton asserts that objectification is in fact necessary for the practitioner to carry out her medical examination. Other medical humanities professors like Rutherford and Maria Vaccarella point out that objectification may be an emotional coping strategy for physicians who may not be receiving adequate mental health support during the course of their duties. One of these distancing strategies is the use of medical jargon and other "objective" language, which can be difficult for the patient to comprehend even in the best of circumstances. Charts, test results, and the labeling of medical records further the sense of depersonalization, as "the 'disembodiment' of the clinical text reaches its limit: the person-as-ill is translated into a series of numbers."[27] This lack of linguistic connectedness is actively redressed in the space of artists' books, where makers appropriate instructional media or verbal commands from healthcare workers that are meant to regulate the patient body. When physicians' words are reprinted in combination with patient narrative, images, and other sensory engagements, new understandings of the impacts of objectivity come into focus.

A text-based artist's book within the Prescriptions Collection from Emma O'Connor, *S:ST298.402*, which is also her assigned patient number, complicates seemingly straightforward exchanges with her physicians by contextualizing their significance against O'Connor's life beyond the hospital doors. Concerning her pre-cancerous genetic testing and the possibility of life-altering stomach removal surgery, O'Connor writes, "the surgeon and his staff were excellent at dealing with the medical aspects of stomach removal but not the family and psychological matters which are important for the rest of your life."[28] These are matters like the guilt her father feels over passing on cancerous genes to his daughter and the socioeconomic factors of healthcare that have impacted her treatment. Even with the promise of future genetic therapies, the artist's book notes that "the financial cost of genetic medicine will result in rationing of public resources, whereas

27 Ibid., 96.

28 Emma O'Connor, *S:ST298.402*, Prescriptions Collection, University of Kent, Canterbury, 2015.

the rich will be able to pay their own way."[29] O'Connor's narrative is an example of how artists' books are able to fill gaps in awareness about the costs of illness, both financial and emotional, from the patient's perspective.

Illness narratives have become an important resource in sociology, psychology, and medical anthropology because of the way they relate illness to subjective bodily experience and the social world of an individual. However, one must ask, "Whose narratives are excluded from the genre because they do not fit within the strict confines of commercial publishing?" Narratives like O'Connor's, which may otherwise be labeled as too short, too personal, or too image-based to be commercially viable, are nevertheless able to gain an audience within a fine arts context. The in-betweenness of book and art is a benefit in this regard. Artists' books do not need to be neat and tidy. In fact, much of their impact comes from the unedited and uncensored testaments of lived experience. As Ducker notes, "the usual mediation of publishing [is] stripped away, and gone with it [are] the modifications of bare, blunt statement into bromides of politeness."[30] The narratives in artists' books can be raw, emotional, immediate, episodic, poetic, mysterious, and unsatisfying, which may ultimately reflect the authentic experience of the illness itself.

While narrativizing an experience of illness has been lauded by many for its positive effects on the sense of agency and meaning-making for the writer,[31] I also argue that the productive tension between that text *in combination with image and materiality* opens the genre of illness narrative to productive abstraction and poetics. Such openness to a subjective interpretation then empowers the reader to also participate in the meaning-making process. This reciprocity between maker and reader increases the potential of establishing intercorporeality. As well, a multitude of writing styles and modes can, as Bolaki states, "create a more inclusive illness narrative canon that de-centers the literary form as the paradigm for understandings of this genre and draws connections between different illness perspectives."[32]

29 Ibid., 30.

30 Johanna Drucker, "Bound to Speak: Accounts of Illness in Artists' Books," *Journal of Medical Humanities* 41, no. 1 (2020): 85.

31 Rita Charon, "Narrative Medicine: A Model for Empathy," *JAMA* 286, no. 15 (2001): 1897–1902.

32 Bolaki, *Illness as Many Narrative*, 3.

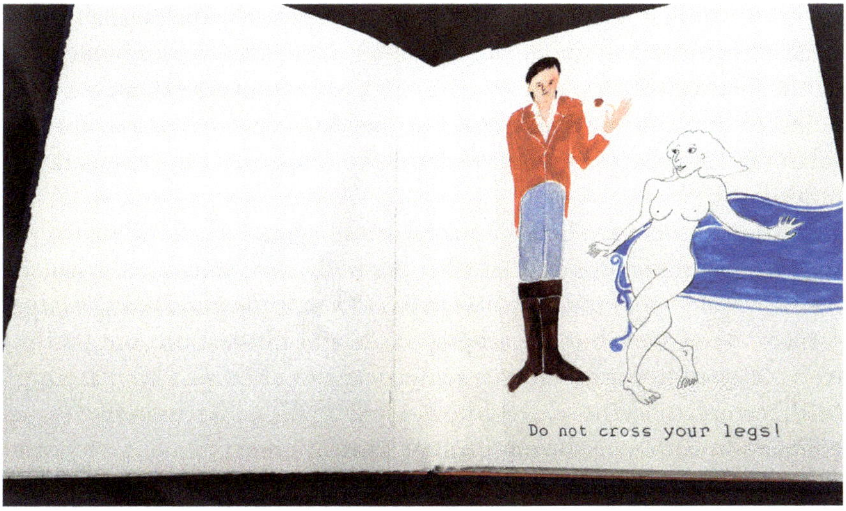

Figure 4.5: Mary Rouncefield, *Mr. Darcy's Advice to the Hip Patient*, Watercolor and ink, 2013.

This inclusivity keeps the medium of artists' books experimental, broadly applied, and resistant to normalization.

A book in the Prescriptions Collection that poetically joins text and image is Mary Rouncefield's satirical *Mr. Darcy's Advice to the Hip Patient* (see Figure 4.5). Rouncefield illustrates a fanciful nude woman flirting with the prim *Pride and Prejudice* character Mr. Darcy across different settings, each in flagrant disregard of the instructions on preventing post-operative hip injury printed at the bottom of the page. Although the woman in the illustrations appears to enjoy breaking the rules, Rouncefield points out the visual metaphors of this figure with regard to her own experience as a hip patient: "The illustrations show the female patient quite naked, emphasizing her complete vulnerability and status as 'patient' and 'victim.'"[33] The nakedness of the female figure compared to the fully suited man also

33 Mary Rouncefield, "Mr. Darcy's Advice to the Hip Patient," in *Prescriptions: Artists' Books on Wellbeing and Medicine*, eds. Stella Bolaki and Egidija Ciricaite (London: Natrix Natrix Press, 2016), 83.

evokes the similar visual trope from the title pages of historical anatomical treatises presented in the previous chapter. Under the veil of humor, the tension between the text and images presented by Rouncefield's artist's book points to the exposure and danger one may feel, especially as a woman, to submit to various states of undress throughout operating and recuperation procedures.

Rouncefield was a bed-bound patient imaginatively fulfilling the desire to do the exact opposite of what her body necessitates and what she has been told (not) to do. *Mr. Darcy's Advice to the Hip Patient*'s larger format, expansive white negative space, bright illustration, and lessons-to-be-learned feel are elements reminiscent of children's books, which further emphasizes the sense of medical paternalism present in the textual commands. Although she must follow "doctor's orders" in order to avoid further injuring herself, her wish for willfulness is safely satisfied within her artist's book.

Re-presenting appropriated text in an artist's book and contextualizing it against imagery and other sensory engagements expands the potential membership to critical medical dialogues, an accessibility consideration that is also present in *Field Notes*. For *Field Notes* in particular, the conversational tone of the text, resulting from piecing together transcripts of my interviews rather than quoting the scholars' published work, avoids overly medical or academic jargon. It may also lower the specialized knowledge necessary for the reader to join the discussion and layer their own views onto the topics brought up. As I will detail in the next section, the same reclamation and gestures toward inclusivity can also be performed for the images of medicine.

Biomedical Images in Artists' Books

Katherine Rawling 38:40

So we've got these historical pictures of patients and their bodies are on display, but we are also understanding them and viewing them as an embodied experience.

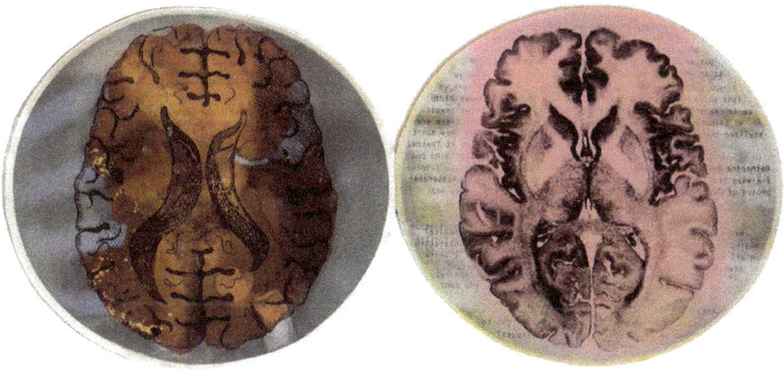

Figure 4.6: Darian Goldin Stahl, *Field Notes: How to Be With*, 2020.

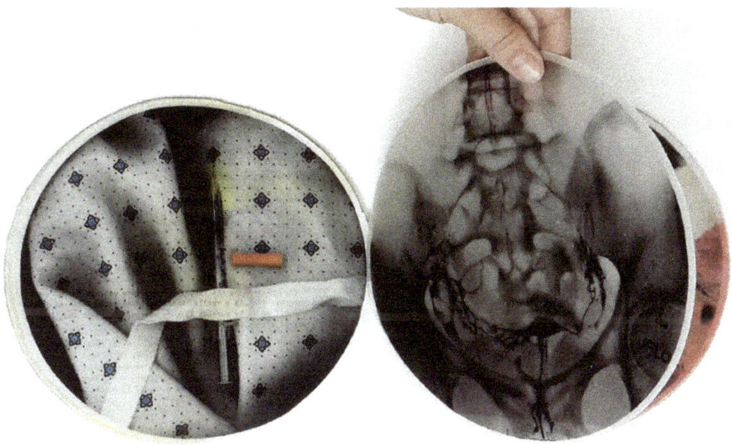

Figure 4.7: Darian Goldin Stahl, *Field Notes: How to Be With*, 2020.

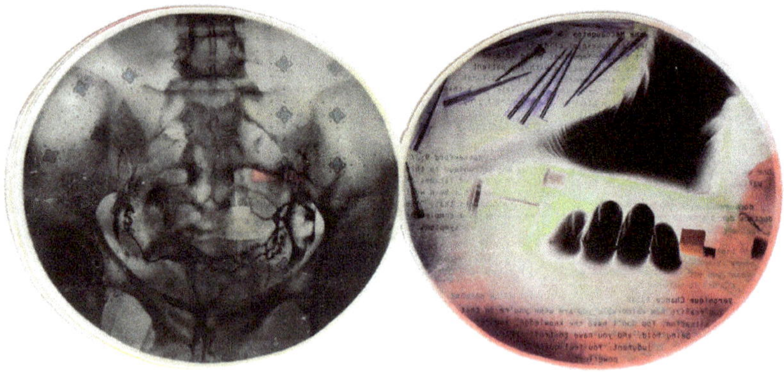

Figure 4.8: Darian Goldin Stahl, *Field Notes: How to Be With*, 2020.

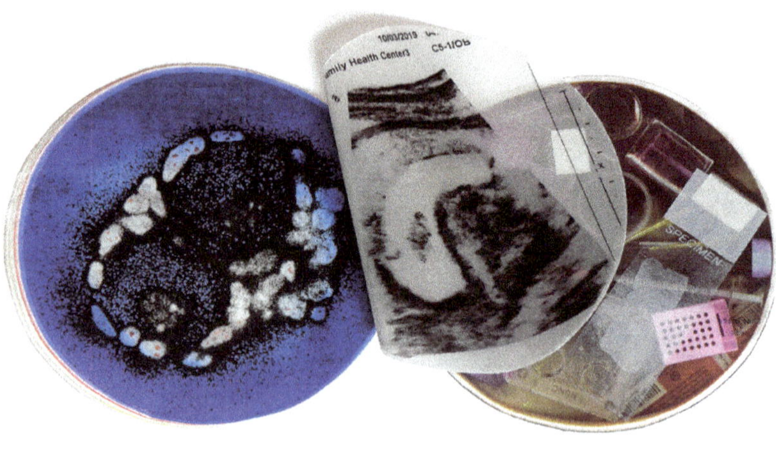

Figure 4.9: Darian Goldin Stahl, *Field Notes: How to Be With*, 2020.

Claire Jones 23:38

We in the history of surgery, of course, we very much look at images. We think about objectivity and think about, actually, that these are stylized—these are in a particular kind of artistic tradition. They don't necessarily represent the body as it looked.

Katherine Rawling 36:03

I always feel a little uncomfortable with people just posting up historical photos of patients.

Fiona Johnstone 21:45

Medical culture is increasingly visual, if you think about medical imaging and also data visualizations. And we are increasingly interested in art-science collaboration and working with visual artists. I think specifically *visual* medical humanities becomes very important.

Katherine Rawling 35:00

Does that mean that we then have the right to do whatever we want with those images?

Jane Macnaughton 13:55

We are, as clinicians and as the general public, charmed by the power of the image. But what we don't understand that I think is extremely complex is the technological processes that have gone into generating that image.

Katherine Rawling 18:09

And this idea of the doctor putting the patient in another uncomfortable or painful position, perhaps a harmful position, just to take a photo? Is that compromising their role as a doctor? But then, are they fulfilling part of the other world of being a doctor by producing medical knowledge?

Rutherford 3:19

Reflect on and consider the possible significance of both the nature of the individual elements contained or recorded within the photograph, and more importantly, their arrangement, composition, or juxtaposition in terms of what that might suggest about things that are of concern to the person who made the photograph.

The objectification patients feel may be no more acute than when physicians gaze upon their medical scans. As Foucault asks in his conception of the medical gaze, "to look in order to know, to show in order to teach, is not this a tacit form of violence, all the more abusive for its silence, upon a sick body that demands to be comforted, not displayed?"[34] Following this thinking, I ask in this section, "If flesh is the site of subjectivity, identity, and the primary medium of engaging and perceiving the world, then what happens to the person's conception of self when her flesh is excised by biomedical imaging technology? How can a physician retain a sense of humanity for her patients when the primary analysis of their bodies is conducted through scans? In the pursuit of visibility, what is subsequently obscured?" Here I explore the consequences of transparency, and how an artistic re-presentation of medical scans in artists' books reclaims a sense of agency over how the body is viewed.

The technological evolution of biomedical imaging has increased the physician's power to represent the entirety of one's illness with a singular scan. With biomedical imaging, one's interiority can now be read and diagnosed far away from the patient's living body. As Leder explains, "the X-ray, MRI, or CT scan results are permanent, reproducible, open to inspection by anyone and everyone, and thus have come to seem the most authoritarian elements of the workup."[35] In light of Foucault's concept of the medical gaze, scholars like Leder, Jackie Stacey, Catherine Haase, and Rosemarie Garland-Thomson further expand on Foucault's notion that an imaged body is a dominated body.

Although patients can be seen as a kind of "collaborator" in the making of biomedical images,[36] a severe hierarchy is emplaced when a patient must submit to the regimes of medicine in order to receive their portrait. Clearing the bowels, fasting, ingesting foul laxatives, or being

34 Michel Foucault, *The Birth of the Clinic* (London: Routledge, 1976), 84.
35 Leder, *The Distressed Body*, 95.
36 Maud Radstake, *Visions of Illness: An Endography of Real-Time Medical Imaging* (Utrecht: Eburon Delft, 2007), 57.

injected with contrast causes considerable discomfort and can be emotionally taxing—not just in the process itself, but also in the anticipation of a diagnosis. All of the biomedical scans included within *Field Notes* originate from Devan's body. MRI scans of her brain (see Figure 4.6), intrauterine fluoroscopy scans (see Figure 4.7), and ultrasounds of her womb (see Figure 4.9) are a visual testament to her long history of submitting to the medical gaze.

The power differentials between the imager and the imaged ensure these seemingly "objective" sights into the body are nevertheless shaped by economic priorities, politics, cultural values, and power. At its worst, one's submission to imaging can be met by those who would take advantage of a patient at her most vulnerable. In Devan's own illness narrative, she recounts such a situation:

> After filling out my preliminary intake forms, I am asked to undress and put on a hospital gown, two if the gown is flimsy. Better safe than sorry. I have found the standards for the clothes I can wear during the exam vary depending on the lab. I once had a rather awkward conversation with a radiology technician about my bra. He was an older, slightly grizzly looking man who introduced himself by asking where I bought my bra. In my vulnerable position, I did not immediately ask why he wanted to know. I assumed he was a professional with a point. Apparently, Victoria Secret bras use a plastic underwire, which is perfectly fine in the MRI scanner. Regardless, he informed me, a metal underwire, like the metal zipper and button on my jeans, would vibrate during the exam, "which some women rather enjoy." This comment left me in the rather awkward position of having to decide whether I should leave my clothes on and allow this man to think I was "enjoying" the exam, or take them off and feel cold for the next two hours.[37]

In addition to this account of sexual harassment, an exchange with Devan's neurologist in the moment of her diagnosis further demonstrates the objectification of Devan's body in the imaging process, albeit in a more covert manner:

> "It's MS!" he declared .... My rather insensitive physician pushed a box of tissues my way without taking his eyes off the computer screen containing my MRI scans. "How can you be sure?" I managed. He looked confused. "I'm not sure what you are

37 Devan Stahl, *Imagining and Imagining Illness* (Eugene: Cascade Books, 2018), 2.

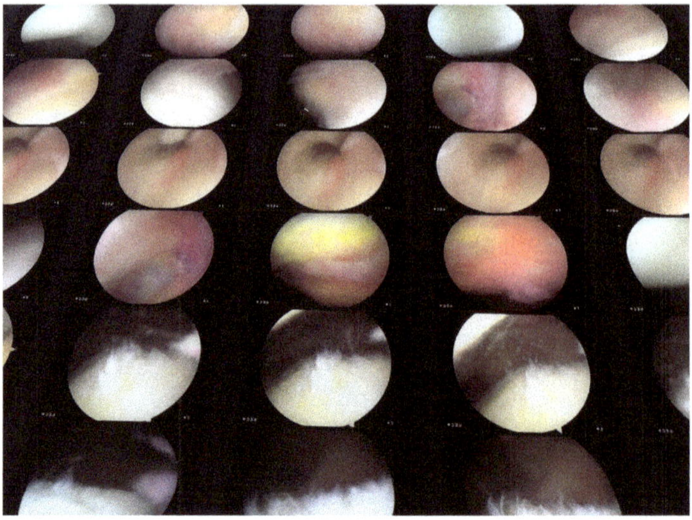

Figure 4.10: Veronique Chance, *In the Absence of Running*, Inkjet on Japanese paper, 2015.

> seeing in those pictures," I followed up. "I'm a specialist" he assured me, in his most proud and patronizing tone. "I know what I am looking for."[38]

Reaching for the chart, avoiding eye contact, and not answering questions reinforce the sense that the images of the body are more useful and important than the patient herself. In her own account of physicians viewing her internal body during the course of treatments, Jackie Stacey also finds that "the copy speaks more urgently and with more authority than the opaque and occluded 'original body.'"[39] The issue of authority, that is, who has the right to capture, print, and interpret internal anatomy, is key to the reclamation of agency experienced by those who appropriate and reprint their imaged body in artists' books.

The power exerted by a medical gaze rooted in patriarchy is exemplified by the Prescriptions Collection artist's book, *In the Absence of Running* by

38 Ibid., 5.

39 Jackie Stacey, *Teratologies* (London: Routledge, 1997), 158.

Veronique Chance (see Figure 4.10). This unbound book consists of two large sheets of paper, about 2 × 4 feet each, which depict a gridded series of round video stills from her arthroscopic knee surgery. In her essay on the making of this book, Chance describes how, although long distance running is a crucial aspect of her healthcare routine and professional career as an artist, her physician did not recommend restorative knee surgery due to her middle age and, Chance suspects, her gender.[40] Chance states, "My experience made me realize how vulnerable one is as a patient and how much those in positions of power can influence decisions and outcomes in treatment."[41] Only after returning to the doctor's office with the support of her male partner was she authorized for surgery.

In *Field Notes*, the vulnerability of the patient's body is most profoundly displayed in Figure 4.7. Here, a cropped view of a hospital gown cradles an orange-capped syringe. On the right-hand side, a pelvis is displayed. A dark substance permeates the center of this anatomy like a drop of ink in water. In reality, this is a fluoroscopy video still of Devan's uterus, which the doctor has injected with contrast to check for blockages in her fallopian tubes that may determine the cause of her infertility. Lifting this page, its transparency causes the reader's hand to become a part of the pelvic composition. On the following spread (see Figure 4.8), a gloved hand grasps a large injection instrument, surrounded by sharp needle caps. These images look scary, invasive, and uncomfortable, and evoke the physical and emotion pain Devan experienced at the time.

Like Chance's arthroscopy stills, Devan's fluoroscopy images are captured in round compositions. And like Chance's images, one may garner many associations from gazing into the body through a dark, circular scope. Looking feels extraordinarily intrusive here, like these images are captured by spying through a door's peephole. The circular view also recalls observing the rodent ovaries through the microscope shown on other pages of *Field Notes,* likening the patient to a specimen. For Chance, the round compositions recall not only "portholes into the body but also a time-sequence of

40 Veronique Chance, "In the Absence of Running: From Injury and Medical Intervention to Art," *Journal of Medical Humanities* 41, no. 1 (2020): 65–80.

41 Ibid., 70.

planets or moons, an abstract painting or a stained-glass window."[42] Finally, the roundness could also recall a telescopic view, securing the notion that the medicalized body can be made present for viewing even from vast distances.

Reclaiming the images of medicine and re-presenting them in artists' books is a strategy for the makers to not only communicate the wider impacts of medical surveillance to their readers but also critique the medical gaze itself through counter-surveillance. Taking medical scans, manipulating them, expanding them, rearranging them, layering them with other images, and reprinting them according to one's own subjective experience of the encounter is an act of defying the submission to medical imagining. Subverting their singular purpose of diagnosis, these now-expansive images make space to express all the ways one's subjectivity was made to feel less-than during their creation.

What were once private and anonymous scans for the sole purview of the medical professional, even out of reach from the patient who had to go through bureaucratic pains to procure them, the artist's bookmaker now wholly determines the view into her body. As an innately shareable medium, artists' books invite readers to view the internal body beneath the flesh of the cover. The *invitation* to look is crucial here, as it flips the conditions of the dominating medical gaze and establishes agency with the maker to determine the parameters of visibility. Instead of gawking or objectifying, readers become ethical viewers in their "capacity to vivify human empathy through bearing visual witness."[43] In the intimate space between reader and book, the artist destabilizes the exclusivity and hierarchies of the medical gaze through the open provocation to reinterpret the imaged body, and entangle all the fleshy and personal impacts surrounding that image.

The readers of *Field Notes* are likewise invited to witness the transformation of medical scans from image to icon, filled with allegory and symbolism of lived experience. As Garland-Thomson explains, "the representational trajectory from Devan as medical specimen—naked before the doctor, entombed in the MRI machine, curled like a fetus on the examining

42 Ibid., 77.

43 Rosemarie Garland-Thomson, *Staring: How We Look* (Oxford, New York: Oxford University Press, 2009), 188.

room floor—to Devan as icon,"[44] is a method for her to view her diseased anatomy as "one she can live in and live with, one that is not broken but beautiful, one fit to behold as a sacred object."[45] For Devan, seeing her body transformed into an artist's book is not only personally meaningful but also exemplifies how the particularities of her experience can grow to encompass multiple subjectivities. She states, "Allowing another person to reshape my body allows me to see the images as universal—they exceed me and invite others to see themselves reflected in [Darian's] art."[46] The intercorporeality of artists' books thus transforms an isolating and vulnerable event into a vehicle for shared understanding and empathy.

Keeping medical images unstable and polymorphic is essential for continually raising new questions about their purposes and impacts. In *Field Notes*, the transparency of Devan's medical scans ensures they are continually complicated by the text and images that appear beneath them and all the unpredictable associations this may hold for the viewer. Even as one lifts the page to view the scans in isolation, the visual presence of the reader's own hand through the transparent page implicates their body in a renewed meaning of this pathology. The essential vitality of artists' books as mediations between embodiments enables a particular diagnosis, like a miscarriage, stomach cancer, knee pain, MS, or infertility, to become part of a network of associations and questions that simultaneously expand and personalize complex meanings of illness.

More-than-Human Bodies in Artists' Books

Whereas the previous sections document the transformation of a patient into a specimen, this section details the transformation of a specimen into

44 Rosemarie Garland-Thomson, "Forward," in *Imaging and Imagining Illness: Becoming Whole in a Broken Body*, ed. Devan Stahl (Eugene: Cascade Books, 2017), xi.

45 Ibid., xii.

46 Stahl, *Imagining and Imagining Illness*, 111–112.

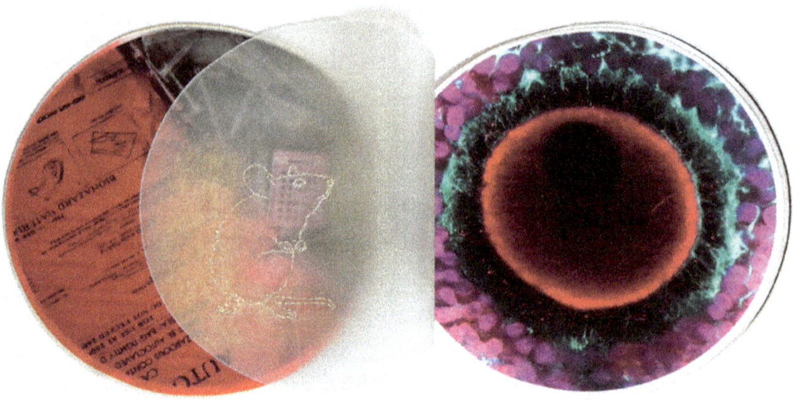

Figure 4.11: Darian Goldin Stahl, *Field Notes: How to Be With*, 2020.

a patient. The use of animal surrogates to stand in for human bodies is a long-standing practice in pursuit of medical progress. Lisa Cartwright likens Foucault's medical gaze to that of scientists gazing into animal anatomy. She states that "the laboratory visual culture is, after all, a culture of human corporeal supervision and discipline, even in cases where the human body is not directly studied … The animal body is a symbolic site where human corporeal regulation is carried out."[47] Imaging isolated specimen organs, like the ovaries and ova from mice printed in *Field Notes*, disguises their animal origins, which makes it all the more palatable to apply the findings of the laboratory onto human bodies.

The most abstract biomedical images in *Field Notes* come from the internal bodies of mice (see Figure 4.11). The frequent presence of stitched rodent bodies and microscopy of their internal structures in this artist's book concerns one of the most controversial subjects in medicine, animal testing. This is a topic that is often overlooked in contemporary health humanities dialogues, whereas the high emotions of conducting research

47 Lisa Cartwright, *Screening the Body: Tracing Medicine's Visual Culture* (Minneapolis: University of Minnesota Press, 1995), 93.

on the ubiquitous dissected bodies of mice was a constant topic of concern with my scientific collaborators in the fertility research laboratory. Animal bodies were broached only once in my twenty-two interviews with health humanities scholars in the UK, from science and technology professor Charlotte Sleigh:

Charlotte Sleigh 17:24
I think one of the interesting challenges is to figure out how we represent interspecies empathy. That is a really important thing to be thinking about, as well. I guess I would be curious to know whether you think that that has any place at all in medical humanities?

Figure 4.11 depicts a stitched outline of a life-sized mouse on a translucent fleshy page in mid-journey across the spine of the book. The thread used to embroider this rodent is gold, and a light wash of gold pigment casts a shadow behind the small mammal. Beneath the mouse on the left-hand page depicts a bright red biohazard bag that includes diagrammatic instructions for properly picking up potentially hazardous materials (like dissected mouse bodies) using the bag. On the right-hand side of this spread is a radiant, technicolor microscopy image of an ovum, consisting of concentric circles and bursts of blues and pinks emanating from a bright red and velvety black center.

The use of gold thread and pigment that outlines the mouse sits against the red warning of the biohazard bag. This placement points to the tension between the mouse being invaluable to scientific research but also disposable once the ova are dissected. Seen in isolation, we are to understand the mouse ova as approximate, even a substitute for, the ova of humans—now made readily available and genetically modified to glow under the microscope's lasers. The radiant microscopy images of the internal structures of ova are almost otherworldly enough to make one forget about the very real bodies put forward as experimental source material. Within the space of *Field Notes*, however, the thickness of the gold thread embosses into the waxed center of the microscopy image of the ovum beneath, ensuring that the mouse's palimpsest remains visible after it's body has been removed. The artist's book's re-contextualization of animal imaging opens the possibility to engage with animal testing in a new way, one where the

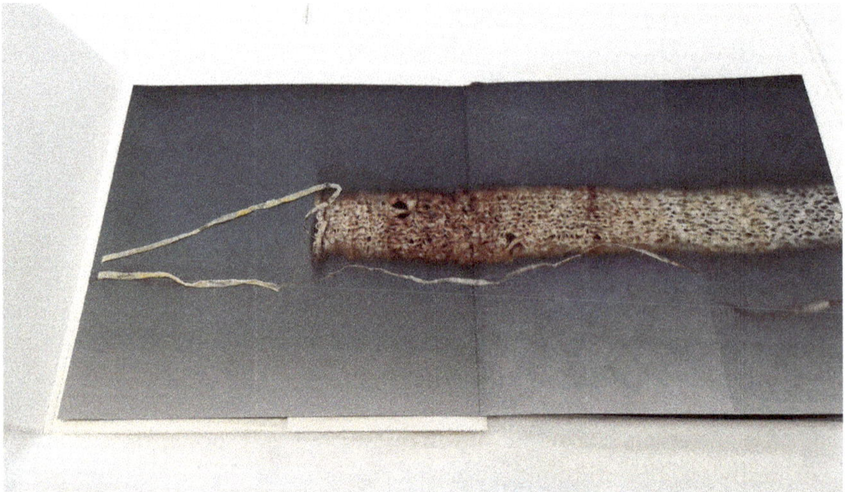

Figure 4.12: Amanda Couch, *Entrail Troyan*, Double-sided inkjet print on variety of Japanese papers and weights, with salami skin collage and threads, bound in 300 gsm. Waterford folio with wax seal, 2016.

care from the researchers and sacrifice of the mice is more openly acknowledged and respected.

Another artist in the Prescriptions Collection who complicates the relation between animal and human bodies in her artist's book is Amanda Couch. Pictured above in Figure 4.12, *Entrail Troyan* depicts a long, knitted tube sculpture that has been Xerox scanned and printed along the length of her concertina book. On the final page, the "thread" used to knit this sculpture leaps off the page and then weaves back through the opposite cover to bind the book together around a puckered red wax seal. This unique seal contains the embossment of the artist's anus.

Couch's article in the *Journal of Medical Humanities* reveals that the sculpture is crafted from knitting together pork sausage casings cut into thin strips so that the sculpture both connotes and is formed with literal entrails.[48] Couch also discloses her struggles with irritable bowel syndrome—a

48 Amanda Couch, "Reflections on Digestions and Other Corporealities in Artists' Books," *Journal of Medical Humanities* 41, no. 1 (2020): 13.

notoriously mysterious condition. Couch fulfills her wish to better understand her vexing guts by materializing them through an animal proxy. Couch uses her "fingers, palms, arms, breasts, legs, wherever a tome was placed, … [to] enact a corporeal connectivity through the haptic."[49] Bowels that are typically hidden in her bodily depths but nevertheless profoundly impact her food and traveling choices can now be engaged with in a way that is meaningful for the author and readers of this artist's book.

The use of animal bodies in art and science continues to draw further parallels to patient experiences. Feelings of being treated "like a lab rat" or "guinea pig" extend the all-too-easy comparisons between the ill and rodents into our common vernacular. In *Field Notes*, the distinctions between animal and human parts are obscured as the book contains microscopy images of *both* human and mouse ova that were used in the scientists' experiments. Without making distinctions between the two, this blending of bodies materializes the extraordinarily complicated issues of consent, ethics, substitution, and innovation when it comes to animal testing. The subsequent goals for raising these controversial issues are to bring attention to the emotional toll of conducting medical research on human and animal bodies, the psychological impacts of oscillating between subjectivity and objectivity for the ill, and finally, the ways an artistic practice can form reflective time and space to consider more-than-human bodies within the realm of the health humanities.

Conclusion: Intertwinings

Melanie Grant 27:16
A lot of "Art in Health" interventions or workshops tend to be quite tokenistic or short lived because there's not much funding for them and they are often seen as secondary to everything else. If we're talking about an ideal future, this approach needs to be valued equally.

49 Ibid., 8.

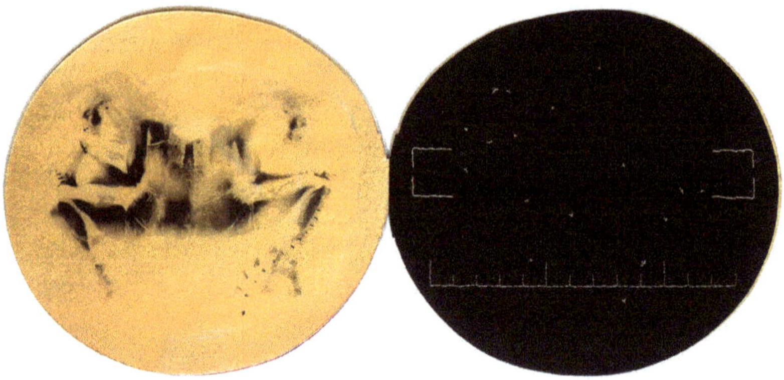

Figure 4.13: Darian Goldin Stahl, *Field Notes: How to Be With*, 2020.

Cathleen Miller 18:54

My feeling is if one or two students are shifted in any way by that experience then it is worth doing.

Charlotte Sleigh 42:19

These things are not easy to do. They take great skill and sensitivity to create a space where people feel safe enough to be in touch with their feelings, their senses, their reactions.

Egidija Ciricaite 17:51

It's impossible to expect every doctor to take very personally, very deeply, every single patient, because there's just no human capacity for that. But this might at least break the cycle of a mechanical approach. It might be something that just stops it for a minute and lets them recharge.

Eleanor Perry: 23:42

It would give them the benefit of being able to utilize these techniques with their patients as a way of getting patients to talk about their embodied experiences, and their psychological experiences, cognitive experiences, neuro-atypicalities—all these kinds of things that are not easy to explain. It would allow them to give patients a means of expression that doesn't rely heavily on language.

Paul Crawford 37:03
I think one of the key strategies, if you're going to be part of the health humanities, is really looking and reflecting upon how you are innovating and building projects "with" not "for."

The final image-based spread shown in Figure 4.13 points to the merger of disciplines in this research-creation outcome. Like the first page of *Field Notes*, the image at the end of the book depicts two bodies next to another microscopic scale, only this time the bodies are merged together around a shared spine. The perceived dualities of art and science, patient and doctor, human and nonhuman, and subjectivity and objectivity are portrayed here as two halves of one body. *Field Notes* fluctuates between ambiguous bodily scales in each spread, slipping between microscopic, internal, animal, human, interpersonal, and population perspectives. The layering of bodies within the intimate, handheld medium counters the growing reliance on technologically mediated screens in order to tangibly connect readers with some of the most critical topics in health humanities. Those texts are then complemented or complicated by the poetic interactions of image and materiality to foster individual significances and manifestations of meaning between the fleshy covers.

The debates raised at the end of *Field Notes* concerning the effectiveness of incorporating artistic practices into the foundations of medical learning is a topic for in the next chapter. In the artist's book itself, there are no final answers to the many debates printed in its pages because the purpose of art, like the practice of phenomenology, is not to instruct but to continually question. The main guidance going forward is provided by health humanities professor Paul Crawford, who encourages a democratic and diverse representation in health humanities scholarship, so that any new pedagogies and practices will be formed " 'with' not 'for.' "[50]

50 Paul Crawford, interview with author, February 26, 2019, in *Field Notes: How to Be With*, ed. Darian Goldin Stahl (2020).

CHAPTER 5

Artists' Books in the Clinic and Classroom

> I make books so I won't die.
>
> —Martha Hall

Introduction

In May of 1989, Martha Hall received a telephone call from a physician she did not know. "'You have breast cancer and you better decide quickly whether you're going to do something about it here [Dartmouth Hitchcock Hospital in Hanover, N.H.] or in Portland [Maine, the nearest major hospital to my home].' With that threat, he hung up."[1] She was 39 years old, had been married for eighteen years, and had two elementary school-aged daughters at the time of this first diagnosis. After studying English at Smith College and receiving a certificate in art education in 1972, Hall made several careers for herself over the subsequent years as an English teacher, weaver, and a weaving supplies small business owner.[2] To expand her marketing skills, she attained an MBA from Dartmouth College in 1989 and transitioned into a career in corporate management. Three years after a second diagnosis of breast cancer, Hall returned to her artistic roots by enrolling in papermaking and bookmaking courses at

1 Martha Hall, "Artist Statement," in *Holding In, Holding On: Artist's Books by Martha A. Hall*, eds. Martha Hall and Martin Antoinette (Northampton: Mortimer Rare Book Room, Smith College, 2003).

2 Maine Women Writers Collection, *Martha A. Hall Collection, 1971–2011*, University of New England, accessed December 18, 2020, <https://library.une.edu/mwwc/collections/collections-a-z/martha-a-hall-collection-1998-2003/>.

Haystack Mountain School of Crafts in Deer Isle, Maine in 1996.[3] This last shift in vocations would ultimately shape Martha Hall's legacy.

After initially deciding not to create art about her diagnosis, poetic text and imagery about living with cancer nevertheless "came to [Hall] spontaneously," and she felt compelled to materialize her long-term illness experiences as artist's books. Hall's artist statement explains that making artist's books "uncovered or *brought to light* emotions [she] had not previously acknowledged. [...] The process of making books has been a powerful part of [her] healing."[4] Hall invested in her arts practice and graduated with a BFA from the Maine College of Art in 1998. After crafting dozens of artists' books about her lived experiences with illness, sharing them with her family and physicians, exhibiting them in galleries across the United States, and depositing them in numerous academic libraries, Hall died from her disease in her beloved home on Orr's Island, Maine, in 2003 at the age of 54. However, Hall ensured her artist's books would continue to speak volumes in her absence. Archived and employed within medical institutions as pedagogical resources, these works continue "to effect change in the way medical professionals interact with their patients."[5]

This chapter follows the unique life of Hall's artist's books: from creation to activation in the clinic, to archive, and finally, to their mobilization in medical classrooms. Throughout this case study, the theme of time plays a dominant role in the lasting impact of Hall's books. Beyond the duration of reading artists' books as a time-based medium, they also engage the concept of time as tools for capturing an event or memory, enduring time in an archive, and resisting the forward momentum of time as capsules of lived experience that persists beyond the author's lifetime. Finally, holding another's autobiographical artist's book transports the reader into a moment in time alongside Hall. Giving space to reflect on the narrative present within artists' books demonstrates that time is the paramount medium of being-with and dignity.

3 Ibid.
4 Hall, "Artist Statement."
5 Ibid.

Medical science is founded upon principles of critique and revision in light of new evidence. Likewise, core values of any committed arts practice are experimentation and evolution. Both science and art persistently apply self-reflexivity to seek out deeper truths about the world in which we operate. However, scientists and artists operate within a particular culture that ultimately shapes the parameters of progress and acceptability, which stymies or propels a sense of shared ethics. While new discoveries can rapidly progress the fields of science, evolving culture (both medical and art) out of harmful biases is a much slower task. It is this culture that artists like Hall hope to influence at the nexus point of patient care.

Employed in the examination room, Hall's artists' books present a destabilizing "flipping of the script" on the typical doctor–patient encounter that may ultimately lead to more productive communication and a sense of holistic care. Within a medical humanities classroom, a thorough investigation of artists' books focuses a reflexive lens onto the systemic injustices of Western medical culture, such as disparate priorities of time, knowledge hierarchies, and a sense of dehumanization. Following Hall's lead, I argue for further integration of the medium into medical humanities pedagogies because artists' books not only give an authoritative account of what it is like to be chronically ill that is otherwise absent from medical textbooks, but they also provoke critical dialogues that scrutinize the Western medical paradigms at the root of patient and practitioner discontents alike.

The Practice of Martha Hall

In contrast with previous chapters, the focus of this investigation into Hall's practice goes beyond the positive impacts bookmaking had on her sense of wellbeing while living under the shadow of cancer for fourteen years. Instead, I center on the unconventional ways she activated her books within the clinical setting as a radical act of self-advocacy. Although Hall initially made books to help communicate with her family, she later "put a huge amount of importance on using the books to communicate with [her] physicians, and [her] nurses, and the medical community in

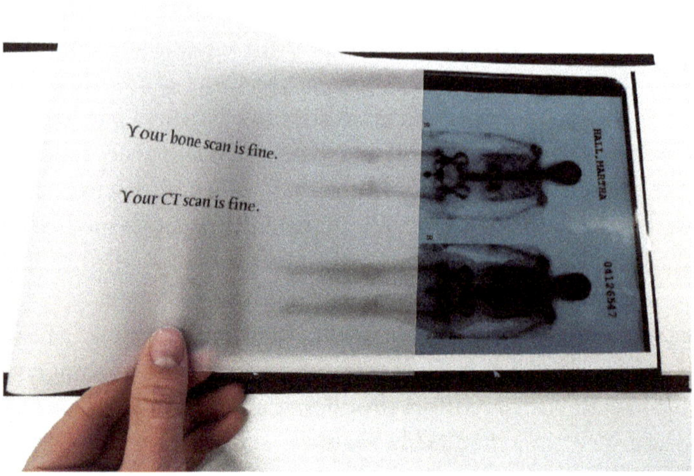

Figure 5.1: Martha Hall, *Voices: Five Doctors Speak*, 1999. This image shows a hand lifting a transparent page of a book with the text, "Your bone scan is fine. Your CT scan is fine." Underneath are two full-body CT scans printed on blue film.

general."[6] Finding success in this endeavor, Hall sought to make her artist's books available to future generations of health professionals within university archives, namely the University of New England, where they could continue to generate vital dialogues around empathy and effective patient care.

One prominent example of Hall's unconventional employment of her artist's books in the clinic is demonstrated within *Voices: Five Doctors Speak* (see Figure 5.1). For this book, Hall transcribed the conversations she had with five of her physicians during an unexpected recurrence of cancer. Each of her physicians is distinguished using a different typeface, although the sentiments they provide are strikingly similar. The first text reads, "Let's find a place to talk," foreshadowing the grim news on the next page that can already be seen through the semi-transparent paper. The following pages

6 Martha Hall, "I Make Books," interview by Jennifer Tuttle, The Maine Women Writers Collection, University of New England, 2004, film, 18:24, <https://www.youtube.com/watch?v=zQCjsutVAtk>.

describe the treatments, side effects she will endure, and a prognosis of living between six months and six years. The final set of translucent vellum pages are glued together to collapse several conversations into a single hazy memory. Through the atmospheric paper, we can just make out the voices describing her treatment, which was not successful: "We failed. You failed."[7] At the end of the book, she writes the names of her doctors using their respective typefaces, as if to credit the coauthors of this moment in her life.

The images in *Voices* include full-body medical scans of Hall that have been re-scanned and scaled to fit within this handheld medium. These images present us with a scan of a scan of Hall, or meta-scan: an image that is reflexive on itself in order to blur the distinctions between observer and subject. The scans appropriated and made into art, along with the transcription of voices from her doctors, turn the tables on who exactly is being examined here.

Hall brought this book into each of her five doctors' offices during her appointments in order to communicate with them how it felt to be diagnosed with cancer again, and how painful it was to hear the words, "You failed." Hall narrates this interaction in the documentary, "I Make Books," which was produced by the University of New England's Maine Women Writers Collection (MWWC) in 2004:

> [Reading from *Voices*] "I didn't want to believe you'd failed. The bone marrow transplant failed. You were responsive to chemo. We failed. You failed." The last thing I want to hear is I "failed." And he was using it in a very medical terminology sense—it meant that, "that treatment failed for you." But it came across as I as a person failed and he as a physician failed. And it wasn't until we really had a chance to talk about that that it softened somewhat for me. But for a long time that, "I failed—We failed" has been a pain.[8]

In another instance, Hall used this book to express her preference for in-person meetings to discuss a diagnosis rather than over the phone:

> [Reading from *Voices*]: "Do you want to speak to me on the phone or in person?" When I sat down with him and we read this page, I said, "That's you. That's what you

7 Martha Hall, *Voices: Five Doctors Speak* (Canterbury: University of Kent, 1999).
8 Hall, "I Make Books."

> said to me." And he goes, "Yeah … so?" And my response was, "It was so important to me to see you in person." And he said, "You don't understand, most people do not want to see me in person. It is too hard to have that difficult emotional time with this person who is somewhat of a stranger. It is very unusual for somebody to want to talk to me in person."[9]

Hall is not questioning the efficacy of her cancer treatments she received, but raising a concern about the other side of practicing medicine. Hall's artist's book initiated a dialogue on the perceived differences in her sense of interpersonal ethics (that cancer diagnoses should be delivered in person) and her physician's past experiences (that most patients prefer to be counseled over the phone). Her physicians also validated the significance of her arts practice by asserting "that the books [she] was creating were more than a form of art therapy and that the books themselves had an intrinsic value."[10] Part of this value was the way in which they helped Hall and her doctors find the common ground to rebuild their relationships going forward.

Although there are clear positive impacts for Hall to activate her artists' books within clinical appointments, one could rightly ask, "Why not just voice these concerns outright? Why go through the trouble of making an artist's book to have this conversation?" First, Hall demonstrates how artists' books can be used as a productive stepping-stone to cross the silence between two people and begin a difficult conversation. Sharing this book as the object of attention surely lifted the pressure of initiating a critique of her physician's language, which may have felt too confrontational otherwise. Next, taking time to make the book away from the stressors of the moment enabled Hall to make herself perfectly clear. Conceiving the book and laboring it into being requires the maker to spend reflective time formulating a response to the perceived slight in a way that feels accurate and assertive. Hall herself recognized that the books were "pushing [her] to communicate a strong message, […] they are a way [she] can have a voice in the world."[11] It is no easy task to question the experience and immense specialized knowledge

9 Ibid.
10 Hall, "Artist Statement."
11 Ibid.

of someone who is charged with saving your life, even when his actions or misconceptions result in distress. Impossible to misread as a passing concern, Hall committed her disquiet to ink, which then became the vehicle to hold and share her truths. Hall's books enabled her to re-orient the agenda of the medical appointment toward her own primary concerns.

I further argue that the authority of well-crafted, hardcover books as cultural icons of knowledge gave Hall the intellectual leverage to broach her concerns with her physicians. It is as if the craftsmanship of the book demonstrates that here is one expert speaking with another expert—leveling a kind of knowledge hierarchy between the two. The imbalance of power and the vulnerability experienced by patients during a clinical encounter is a vital motivation for bookmakers to rearrange expressive authority. The physician demonstrates their expertise through the accurate interpretation of tests and scans, providing a cogent diagnosis, and formulating a treatment plan, and the patient is typically the passive recipient of such knowledge. In Hall's case, she was also able to demonstrate an expertise over her own lived experiences of illness by seizing the authority of the book. In sharing these artist's books with her doctors, Hall provides the material to be discussed, rich with metaphor, sensory expressiveness, and inclusive of the impacts of disease that fall outside of the strict delineations of the personal and the medical, such as the impact of doctor–patient relationships and her sense of wellbeing. Artists' books in the clinical encounter thus shift a study of the body to a study of embodiment.

Artists' books are probably something very new for the physician, and any subsequent uncertainty they evoke is key to opening the imagination and understanding his patient's particularities anew. Like the practice of phenomenology, Hall's books prompt her physicians to reassess their habituated responses to what are, for them, common situations of delivering bad news. Hall recounts that being confronted with their own voices in her artist's book "elicited responses of denial, disbelief, discomfort"[12] from her doctors. Provoking a slight sense of discomfort in an unexpected artist's book intervention pressed the physicians to hear their own voices anew and reassess the impact of those word choices. Taking the time to read this

12 Ibid.

book together provided Hall's physicians with more insight into her experiences, and they were then able to become better partners in her care. Although the progression of her cancer was out of her control, Hall was able to redirect this aspect of her treatment. Thus, the greatest outcome of Hall's interventions was to rebalance her relationships with her physicians and bend the clinical appointment toward what they could accomplish together. Within an unstructured meeting over an artist's book, agendas are set aside, unanticipated insights emerge, and being-with becomes possible.

In the final pages of *Voices*, there is a much smaller book tucked into a pocket. It is titled *Legacy*, and it depicts joyous dancing skeletons and a conversation with one doctor about the contrast between her terminal diagnosis and the lasting impact of her books. This small book foreshadows Hall's wish that her books continue to promote patient empathy in her absence, even after her death, by archiving her creations and integrating them into medical education.

Mobilizing Hall's Artist's Books in Medical Humanities Pedagogies

The second life of Hall's books began after medical institutions across the US and UK, including Dartmouth, Smith, and Wellesley Colleges, Harvard University, and the University of Kent acquired these works. The largest collection of Hall's artist's books resides with the University of New England's Maine Women Writers Collection (MWWC). Hall wanted her books in these archives because she thought they would be able to reach her target audiences of medical learners, researchers, and practitioners. The head outreach archivist for the MWWC, Cathleen Miller, attests that "by providing wide access to Hall's artist's books in both the classroom and the archives, the MWWC has answered Hall's call for conversation and consciousness-raising among current and future healthcare providers."[13] I conducted archive fieldwork at the MWWC

13 Cathleen Miller and Jennifer Tuttle, "'I make books so I won't die': Artists' Books in the Archives and in the Classroom," in *Prescriptions: Artists' Books on Wellbeing*

and the University of Kent and interviewed their respective librarians in order to witness the fruition of Hall's legacy. I wanted to experience the books firsthand and learn about the special considerations of archiving such unusual books, the librarians' own efforts to integrate them into coursework, and the reactions they witness from the students who engage with them.

As a part of university archives, medical humanities instructors have the opportunity to mobilize Hall's artists' books in the classroom. The goals for integrating arts-led[14] pedagogies in medicine are diverse, and include increased comfort with ambiguity, observation and communication skills, and fostering empathy. While these qualities are important, a focus on the utility of medical humanities to improve physician's hard and soft skills risks neglecting the ways humanities methodologies can formulate criticality around more systemic issues in the institution of medicine. A more critical wave of medical humanities scrutinizes the peripheral instrumentalization of the arts to "soften the edges" of medicine rather than their potentiality to create time, space, and permission for a reflexive critique of medicine's cultural paradigms. Medical ethics and philosophy professor Jeffery Bishop's provocatively titled essay, "Rejecting Medical Humanism," calls out what he deems to be superficial medical humanities pedagogies that merely obscure the hierarchies of power within medicine without taking measures to dismantle them.[15] Bishop argues that it is only when physicians forgo the push for efficiency, reclaim the time of being-with patients, and invite those with lived experiences of illness to become co-creators of healthcare knowledge that the medical humanities will succeed.

The *critical medical humanities* has emerged in the past decade within the UK to meet such aims, and begins with the conclusion that the medical humanities are not consequential enough to instigate the paradigm changes needed to achieve healthcare equity. Rather than setting therapeutic goals

---

and Medicine, eds. Stella Bolaki and Egidija Ciricaite (London: Natrix Natrix Press, 2017), 11.

14 "Arts-led" pedagogies connotes studying artworks as research material, not necessarily making new artworks.

15 Jeff Bishop, "Rejecting Medical Humanism: Medical Humanities and the Metaphysics of Medicine," *The Journal of Medical Humanities* 29 (2008): 22.

for medical students by practicing the arts and humanities, like elective creative writing courses aimed at alleviating stress and burnout, this more critical perspective challenges the institution to investigate the reasons why so many students experience burnout in the first place and then remodel such harmful learning environments. A proposed method for such a reevaluation is to work with arts and humanities practitioners toward a common ethics of care for one another. This requires institutions to integrate arts and humanities methodologies based on feminist, disability, race, queer, and decolonial theories expressed through variable modalities like art and research-creation. Working together, the critical medical humanities can become a shifting and progressive pedagogical space, challenged to consistently reevaluate the practices and teaching of medicine to meet the evolving needs of students, patients, and practitioners.

Failure to address harmful institutional paradigms has dire effects on students. M. L. Jennings reports that "the epidemic of medical student burnout can be attributed to a technocratic paradigm that fails to value medical students as persons with human needs and limitations."[16] The suppression of natural emotion, overwhelming workloads, and push for more technologically mediated ways of interacting with patients are all found to cause feelings of detachment, which result in "elevated rates of depression, anxiety, suicidal ideation, and overall poor mental health as compared to themselves at matriculation and to their age-matched peers."[17] A strong rationale for integrating the humanities in healthcare is to carve out time, seemingly inefficient time, within the demanding pace of medicine to practice being-with. I posit that spending time with first-person artists' books, hearing their stories, allowing oneself to feel the emotions they bring up, and engaging the sensing body as a co-creator of their meanings is a potentially transformative practice to counter the depersonalizing effects of studying and practicing medicine.

Critical medical humanities proponents out of the University of Durham, like Jane Macnaughton, Havi Carel, and Angela Woods, question

16 M. L. Jennings, "Medical Student Burnout: Interdisciplinary Exploration and Analysis," *Journal of Medical Humanities* 30 (2009): 253.

17 Ibid., 253.

the kinds of narrow modalities that are typically employed in medical humanities classrooms, which are currently dominated by the study of Narrative Medicine.[18] While giving full credit to Rita Charon and her concept of Narrative Medicine[19] for constructing a lasting bridge between medicine and the humanities, an inclusive approach to being with the stories and experiences of others must acknowledge that certain experiences are too overwhelming, too taboo, or too visual for narrative to capture alone.[20] The task of formulating the events of your life into a coherent narrative may prove to be an insurmountable barrier for some. To help fill the epistemic gap, University of New England medical humanities and English professor Jennifer S. Tuttle partners with librarian Cathleen Miller to teach health science students about patient experiences by mobilizing Hall's artist's books. These reflexive, multi-sensory artworks ignite a dialogue on systemic concerns in Western medicine, most notably, the hierarchies between doctors and patients, managed time, and the suppression of emotion.

Hierarchies

Although there are numerous forms of hierarchies that can be found within medicine, for this discussion around artists' books, I will focus on the disparities between expert medical language and the patient's attempts to communicate her own lived experience. Such disparities in knowledge and language may ultimately construct barriers, confusion, and distrust in doctor–patient relationships. Hall writes that the "mysterious language of medicine" left her frustrated and angry, which she expressed in her artist's books as "terse sentences, irony, humor, color, [and] images that cannot be understood."[21] Havi Carel explains that the perceived status of being able to accurately recount one's symptoms that

18 Angela Woods, "The Limits of Narrative: Provocations for the Medical Humanities," *Medical Humanities* 37, no. 2 (2011): 76.

19 Rita Charon, *Narrative Medicine: Honoring the Stories of Medicine* (Oxford: Oxford University Press, 2008).

20 Bishop, "Rejecting Medical Humanism," 22.

21 Hall, "Artist Statement."

conforms to medical terminology can lead to a form of epistemic injustice, wherein the patient is at a disadvantage in articulating their experiences.[22] For example, if an ill person improperly applies medical jargon, "they are often regarded as cognitively unreliable, emotionally compromised, or existentially suspect."[23] This injustice is also confirmed in artist Christina Lammer's experience of documenting radiology technicians, who privately mock a patient's misuse of medical language, because, Lammer suspects, "the patient's attempt to make him/herself understood is seen as a foreign intrusion into the language of medical expertise."[24] To right this injustice, patients must be seen as the experts of their own experiences, and deference must be applied to meet ill persons where they are and the types of communication they employ.

The authority engendered by a printed and bound book gives tacit credence to the patient's testimony inside. A close read of Hall's artist's books by medical students repositions her from a *medical* non-expert to a primary resource of *illness* knowledge in ways that are novel, expansive, and meaningful. Although medical humanities students regularly engage with patients recounting their symptoms through narrative readings or case studies, they are rarely afforded such an intimate, multi-sensory experience of how encompassing and world-altering illness can be. Released from narrative, artists' books use the aspects of bookness to tangibly show readers how illness causes a "global sense of disorder" that may inhibit the patient's ability to effectively communicate.[25] Hall's books provide a glimpse into this other world.

Although Hall achieved a high level of education and even many years of English teaching experience, changes to her sense of global order during

22 Havi Carel, *The Phenomenology of Illness* (Oxford: Oxford University Press, 2016), 183.

23 Ibid., 182.

24 Christina Lammer, "Bodywork: Social Somatic Interventions in the Operating Theaters of Invasive Radiology," in *Visual Interventions: Applied Visual Anthropology*, ed. Sarah Pink (Oxford: Berghahn, 2007), 128–129.

25 S. Kay Toombs, "The Body in Multiple Sclerosis: A Patient Perspective," in *The Body in Medical Thought and Practice*, ed. Drew Leder (London: Kluwer Academic Publishers, 199), 134.

acute periods of her cancer treatments caused Hall to have mental confusion and verbal incoherence. She encapsulates this unsettling experience in her artist's book, *Prescriptions*. In it, Hall writes, "The pharmacist always asks if I have any questions and I always say no." This response is then immediately contradicted with numerous lingering questions on the following pages:

> Why is my oncologist so quick to prescribe a drug? Might there not be something that I am doing or eating or not doing or not eating that I could change? How long did I need to wait to see if the first pills worked? And what if they don't? What was the next prescription to try? How long did I need to wait and see if this one worked?[26]

She goes on to explain that the twenty-two medications prescribed during this round of cancer treatment, scanned and reprinted into this book, inhibit her ability to respond to her pharmacists' hurried questions. Hall writes that she will "wake up with a foggy brain," a feeling that is visually conveyed to the reader as the semi-transparent pages form a foggy atmosphere over her texts. Tuttle and Miller attest that this book is "humbling for such readers, demanding that they listen to reticence as well as honor questions, using their imagination and empathy in unexpected ways"[27] in order to anticipate their patient's unspoken concerns.

A reflexive engagement with artists' books has the potential to alert the reader to the epistemic injustices, like those expressed in Hall's artwork, and ultimately, apply more accommodating communications with their own patients. To apply such self-critique, Carel attests that the onus of communication is on the physician, not the patient. She prescribes medical professionals to think, "the fact that I don't understand you is not your fault but mine; even your best efforts to make yourself understood are failing, not because of their inarticulacy, but because I am untrained in the appreciation of the sort of articulacy you are using, and this hermeneutical context does not provide me with those resources."[28] The value of Hall's books in this teaching context is to promote entry points into a

26 Martha Hall, *Prescriptions*, Maine Women Writers Collection, Portland.

27 Jennifer S. Tuttle and Cathleen Miller, "Unruly Voices: Artists' Books and Humanities Archives in Health Professions Education," *Journal of Medical Humanities* 41, no. 1 (2020): 57–58.

28 Carel, *The Phenomenology of Illness*, 188.

reflexive dialogue over which modes of expressions we deem valid and useful, and how to meet others where they are. It is only within this emotional and intellectual work, prompted by the subtle forms of bookness and meaning-making communicated in Hall's work that do not only rely on words, that the hierarchies between medical and patient communication can begin to be leveled.

Making Time

Perhaps the greatest change to Hall's global sense of order during her cancer treatment was the total management of her time. Hall's artist's book, *The Rest of My Life II*, palpably displays how cancer and its treatments overtake every other priority of how to spend time (see Figure 5.2). To create this book, Hall collected every medical appointment card and small prescription envelope she was given over the course of one year and sewed this medical ephemera loosely together end-to-end. The address, date, and time for each appointment are printed on the front, and a fragmented accounting of her decade-long illness narrative is handwritten across the back of these cards:

> April 1989. I found a lump in my left breast.// May 1989. I was diagnosed with stage one breast cancer.// July through September 1993. Hospitalized at Maine Medical Center for three rounds, high dose chemo.// September 1999. Cancer in my hips, spine, skull, ribs and liver.[29]

Hall also records more personal dates that were impacted by her intense treatment schedule: "August 1993. I missed our family reunion."[30] Finally, Hall projects time into the future tense: "No urn. Wood box. Plant elm tree or lupine field. Party. No organ donation. If any money Haystack or Navajo Nation scholarships to first-third grades."[31] Although Hall's text reveals the gravity of her illness, it is the sheer number of appointment cards

29 Martha Hall, *The Rest of My Life II*, Maine Women Writers Collection, 2000.
30 Ibid.
31 Ibid.

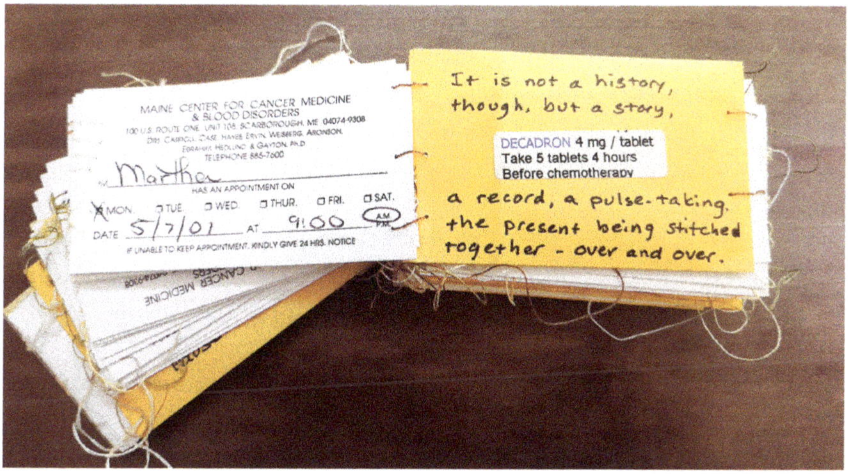

Figure 5.2: Martha Hall, *The Rest of My Life II*, 2000. This image shows a stack of medical appointment cards that have been loosely sewn together into a concertina book. The left-hand page gives Hall's appointment information, and the right-hand page is a small envelope that once held a dose of medication. On this envelope, Hall as written, "It is not a history, though, but a story, a record, a pulse-taking, the present being stitched together—over and over."

that lends this book its expressive heft. Holding them stacked together, one can literally feel the cumulative impact of illness and its domination over how time is controlled by medical treatments. *The Rest of My Life II* collapses past, present, and future into a tangible weight.

Reclaiming these cards and choosing to spend her time transforming them into book pages enables Hall to gain back some authority over her regulated body and the goals for the time she had left. Such arts interventions challenge where time should be spent as one nears the end of her life. Hall writes that "the themes are universal and speak to family, friends and strangers living with the fear of dying in order to live, creating to heal myself and others, leaving a legacy, appreciating and living fully each day."[32] By binding together the printed ephemera that recorded her location on any

32 Hall, "Artist Statement."

given day, who she saw, and how she felt, Hall transformed her terminal embodiment into something permanent.

In my interview with Miller over how she mobilizes Hall's books in the classroom, she explains that *The Rest of My Life II* "has a lot of impact for students" because of the realization that this tall stack of cards "is only a tiny portion of what she actually experienced."[33] What makes Hall's books successful for learning about the patient's experience of time is the phenomenological transformation of habituated ephemera into something iconic. Clinical appointment cards are a ubiquitous tool of regulating time and ensuring an uninterrupted schedule; but in her appropriation of these cards for an artist's book, Hall morphs the everyday into the daunting prospect of being ill every day and all of the physical and emotional demands of such frequent hospital visits. Hall's manipulation of the familiar requires readers to stop, take notice, and experience the affect of these cards from her particular point of view. In her invitation to hold and read this book, Hall exchanges the control over her time for that of the readers'—commanding their time to reflect on her illness.

It is no wonder that one of the most impactful aspects of artists' books is in their capacity as a time-based medium. Medical students are likely to identify with the total management of their time by the institution of medicine, such as set course schedules, heavy rotation itineraries, and eventually long stretches of time on call. Twenty years after her passing, Hall's books continue to promote a common ground between the patient's sense of ethics and the demands of practicing medicine. After studying Hall's books, Tuttle and Miller invite the medical students to respond to Hall's critiques of an apparent lack of holistic care that results from such quick and frequent medical appointments. The instructors report that the "students did empathize … and acknowledge the challenges she faced as a patient, but they also wanted the patient to understand just how difficult it was for them to offer the rigorous, thoughtful, attentive care most beneficial for the patient in the span of time allotted by our healthcare system."[34] These reflections highlight that in a healthcare system that places upmost value

33 Cathleen Miller, interview by Darian Goldin Stahl, July 29, 2019.

34 Tuttle and Miller, "Unruly Voices," 61.

on efficiency, the dizzying speed of face-to-face time between doctors and their patients can leave both parties wanting.

The tensions caused by tight clinical schedules is a discrepancy between feelings of what Arthur Frank terms as "rightness," or the identification of what is ethical and proper by particular agents within a particular space.[35] For physicians, temporal rightness generally revolves around how many patients they can see and treat in a day. For the patients, rightness may mean taking the time to fully explain potential diagnoses, recounting the impacts of illness on their lives, or assessing how potential treatments fit within their ideas of living well. Both parties feel that their expectations for rightness are being compromised by the other. The differences of temporal rightness make the patient feel as though her (dis)comfort is unconsidered or that her emotions are not as important to staying on schedule. In giving primary attention to turnover instead of spending the time necessary for the patient in the room to cover all of her spoken and unspoken questions, that is, "to see certain collateral damage as right,"[36] reveals the depersonalizing systems and pressures in which physicians are trained.

The disparity of temporal expectations between a patient's ethics of care, or even politeness, and the pressure for clinical efficiency is a systemic cause for much of the dissatisfaction within patient and doctor interactions. Such discrepancies of rightness are already apparent in this chapter through Hall's account of the pressures she felt to not take up too much time. Either from the vaguely threatening command that she "better decide quickly" where to receive her cancer treatment, her physician's suggestion of relaying her diagnosis over the phone, or the pharmacist rushing past her potential questions, the speed of medicine is shown to be misaligned with the priorities and abilities of the ill person.

By creating space for meditative reflection in the making and reading of her artist's books, Hall resists the pressures for speed. Perhaps Hall's most profound act of countering the efficiency of medicine was to insist

35 Arthur Frank, "Rightness, Place, and Humanistic Health Care Ethics: Fragments of a Moral Inquiry," *GeoHumanities* 4 (2018): 310.

36 Ibid., 312.

that her physicians take the time to read her artist's books with her. Hall recounts such a demand with a reluctant physician in her documentary:

> He was the one who had not seen this book. I would bring it in from time to time and he would say, "I don't have time. I don't have this; I don't have that." There was one day when he came in and I said, "I am going to be giving a talk on my books, and somebody is going to ask me, because they always do, 'Have all the doctors seen this book?' And I am going to say, 'No. The one who was most black and white and the one who I was most angry at has not seen it.' And I still have this anger because you won't look at it. And I am going to tell them that you have not looked at it." He said, "Alright. Alright. I will look at it." So he is sitting in his chair, and I am sitting in mine, and we are way too far apart. He is on that side of the little room and I am on this side of the little room. And I said, "If you are going to look at it, let's move your chair and I will move my chair and you are going to sit next to me. And you are going to look at it." And we did.[37]

Moving from behind his desk, forgoing the schedule, and spending time *alongside* Hall demonstrate how arts interventions can begin to realign the sense of rightness between doctors and patients.

In Miller and Tuttle's medical humanities classes, taking the time to attentively read Hall's artist's books provides students with a reprieve from the systemic pressures of clinical efficiency, at least for a while. As they collectively discuss Hall's artwork and write thoughtful responses to Hall and her family, these students are learning how to honor the experiences of the subject through close listening and giving her their time. When the currency of dignity is time, providing the space for durational being-with is imperative to countering the emotional tolls of practicing medicine.

The Suppression of Emotion

In his case for integrating the humanities into medical education, Bleakley attests that systemic insensibility within Western medical practice results in a spectrum of injustices, which "includes the objectifying of patients, teaching by ritual humiliation, empathy decline, emotional

37 Hall, "I Make Books."

over-insulation, moral erosion and cynicism, intolerance of ambiguity, paternalism, poor self-care and heroic individualism, all of which can lead to medical error."[38] Jennings also finds that the "suppression of natural emotions on the wards" contributes to the pressure to exhibit stoic detachment. "A medical culture which defines its physicians as heroic and invincible cannot even 'conceptualize' a need for physician and student self-care."[39] Compounding these issues, the depersonalization felt by patients within a profit-driven care system can be felt equally by the physicians, as "the sheer overwork and constant stress, giving rise to exhaustion, anxiety, pressure, and resentment, may make the new hospital admission seem more like the 'enemy' than a focus for one's compassionate care."[40] Not providing the space to express or reflect on the inherent emotions of a job as perilous as medicine is antithetical to health and wellbeing. While Hall and the artists discussed in the previous chapter employ artists' books to reclaim a sense of emotional care for themselves, the rest of this chapter will investigate how arts-led practices make space and give permission to medical students to share in the emotions these artists' books evoke.

While mobilizing Hall's artist's books in the classroom, Miller recounts that the heavy topics of illness and dying enabled the students to broach emotions within a constructive, low-stakes environment: "There are some students who have been personally touched by cancer in their lives in a close way, and those students connect with the narrative really intensely and emotionally. That anger and the frustration and the things that we're taught to shove down and put away and not show other people, I think there's something really powerful in that for students to see—to see that expression of things that are usually forbidden."[41] Joanna Baines, librarian at the University of Kent, additionally attests that the strong emotional impact of artists' books lies in their multi-sensory expression

38 Alan Bleakley, "When I Say … The Medical Humanities in Medical Education," *Medical Education* 49 (2015): 960.

39 Jennings, "Medical Student Burnout," 250.

40 Drew Leder, "Introduction: The Body in Medical Thought and Practice," *Philosophy and Medicine* 43 (1992): 7.

41 Miller, interview.

of illness, which is "very different to just reading a book about it … you can't *not* engage with it."[42] The intimacy of holding an artist's book close to the body and activating our senses to understand its meaning make this art form especially emotive.

In my time in the archives, I found that handling these books was far more affective than I had even anticipated. I had already read Hall's statements and watched her documentary, but *touching* these books engaged a level of emotion that had remained untapped before this moment. It was as if these books were a time machine or talisman that transported me alongside Hall to bear witness to all the anger, sadness, and love motivating these works. The feeling that this object was carefully crafted by the hands of a person who died, who had so little time left but chose to spend it making this object for *you* to experience and learn from, imbues every page with affect. The relationality felt in these auratic objects gives them a power to evoke compassion and empathy through time, distance, and even mortal planes.

I further posit that employing Hall's books within medical learning provides an object of attention—a kind of emotional lightening rod—to initiate productive group discussions and private reflections on the emotional tolls of medicine. Rather than being prompted to speak toward one's own past experiences, which may be too personal or seen as unprofessional in a classroom setting, a focus on the numerous complex facets of illness that are contained within Hall's books enables a dialogue around emotions that they may not have been comfortable breaching otherwise. Tuttle and Miller have found that their students ultimately "articulate their thanks for having found in her books a secure place to speak openly about mortality."[43] Mobilizing Hall's artist's books as stepping stones toward more open and honest discussions about medicine was precisely the kind of communication Hall was hoping to provoke when she donated her books to medical archives.

Nevertheless, holding artists' books and experiencing their uneasy stories can be upsetting. Hall acknowledges the emotional impact her books

42 Joanna Baines, interview by Darian Goldin Stahl, January 31, 2019.
43 Tuttle and Miller, "Unruly Voices," 59.

will have on future readers. She states, "People may not want to 'touch' the topics I explore in my books; yet the books invite handling, touching, interactions."[44] Hall hints at the promotion of empathy inherent in experiencing another's artist's book because "they compel not only physical involvement with the book, but also involvement with the ideas expressed in the art and text."[45] This level of discomfort and vulnerability may be more than readers are willing to handle. Therefore, librarian Joanna Baines, who also mobilizes Hall's books in her pedagogies, insists that medical humanities instructors and facilitators must be especially attuned to the emotional states of their students. When she encounters particularly affective reactions, Baines uses this opportunity to form a self-reflective call and response:

> Let's talk about this reaction. Let's talk about what this means. Why do you feel like that? What is it that's freaking you out? … When you're looking at material, when you're looking at the physicality of an object, think about those reactions. They are important, and they're valid.[46]

This kind of inquisitive care normalizes the presence of emotions surrounding topics of illness and how to respond productively, which may then go on to unseat bias and aversion against natural empathetic responses.

The articulations of meaning-making evoked through Hall's books are further cemented by Tuttle's responsive coursework assignments. Tuttle requires students to write essays on the themes presented in Hall's books, as well as compose response letters to Hall's surviving family that they may choose to mail. The opportunity for written reflection gives students who may be reluctant to engage in open dialogue the chance to thoroughly review their experiences. Tuttle explains that the "students' letters make clear the emotional and affective impact of Hall's work and allow future healthcare practitioners to enact the kinds of listening and dialogue that Hall so fervently sought."[47] These letters exemplify how informal or private

44 Hall, "Artist Statement."
45 Ibid.
46 Baines, interview.
47 Tuttle and Miller, "Unruly Voices," 58.

writing can be a productive method of processing emotionally challenging situations for the students. Mindful, creative, and time-intensive practices give permission for medical practitioners and learners to slow down, reflect, and reacquaint oneself with the sensing body—a practice which may ultimately aid in sustaining wellbeing and humanity in their clinical practices.

Tuttle and Miller's sustained teaching and publishing collaboration in the pursuit of integrated medical humanities pedagogies also demonstrates the productivity of co-teaching to dismantle disciplinary hierarchies. Their expertise of the subject matters and theoretically grounded pedagogies are essential for constructing courses that foster productive reflexivity and increase the chance of student buy-in. The students in these courses are able to practice being-with and fostering empathy in a supportive environment, which evidences the intrinsic transformative potential of arts-led research. Miller attests that Hall's books have been overwhelmingly successful as primary resources of illness experiences and instigating reflexive dialogue around better patient care. Ultimately, this work honors Martha Hall and the efforts she made to materialize and archive the legacy of her life. The institutional investment in artists' books may also feel like the makers' labor, point of view, and even their lives have been given value. As Hall states,

> In leaving a legacy, they are helping me to feel that my life has value. [...] What makes me feel like all that I do has value is knowing that there will be some students who are going to be pursuing medical careers, in the medical profession in one way or another, who will have access to these books and will have a way to react to them.[48]

Conclusion

Spending time engaging with patient-made artists' books in the clinic or classroom is a practice of giving dignity the subject. These works in turn provide an invitation for readers to reflect on what it means to be ill and live well. Not all doctors will be willing to put aside their agenda for

48 Hall, "I Make Books."

the examination, and not all patients desire to make art or express their vulnerabilities. However, Hall's bookmaking practice exhibits a kind of holistic caretaking that was fostered alongside her physicians. There was ultimately no permanent recovery from Hall's cancer, but by taking the time to sit and be with Hall, to pour over her books together, and to change their own communication practices based on the critiques presented in her artwork, Hall's physicians provided the care she required.

Inviting critique on the emotional, temporal, and hierarchical facets of medicine may feel uncomfortable and disruptive, but may nevertheless instigate the reflexivity required to imagine new ways of teaching and practicing medicine. In donating her artists' books to an archive, Hall hoped to provoke more critique and dialogue about what it is like to move through the Western medical system with future generations of doctors. In Hall's words, "My hope in the long run would be that if something is meaningful to someone, or they learn something, or they have a perspective that is different from mine … I would hope that from time to time, somebody would carry on another piece of the conversation."[49] Artists' books' sensory and textual expressiveness, duration, and intimacy make this medium uniquely suited to provoke such dialogues, and ultimately form the relationality necessary for physicians and patients to work together as partners toward wellbeing.

49 Ibid.

CHAPTER 6

"Book as Body" Workshops: A Case Study of Health Humanities Pedagogies

Introduction

Beyond the comprehension of lived experiences evoked by reading another artist's book, I aim to discover what embodied insights health and medical learners gain by making their own artists' books on illness. To this end, I designed and conducted health humanities workshops that teach participants about the historical intersections of books and bodies, how to read contemporary artists' books on illness, and finally, the guidance and know-how to create their very own artists' books. This chapter focuses on the formation and outcomes of these "Book as Body" workshops as case studies for the potentiality of research-creation within health humanities context. The data collected from the workshops are then used to analyze how the collective creation of artists' books might promote relationality around themes of illness and medicine.

This analysis is meant to be a philosophical rationale and pragmatic example for those interested in artist-led, collaborative, or co-taught health humanities pedagogies. During my investigations in health humanities, I found a dearth of art-making pedagogies in comparison to other methods like Narrative Medicine, museum visits, and theater.[1] Even Tuttle and Miller's medical and health humanities courses reflect on Hall's books primarily through writing, and not necessarily by making artists' books for themselves. Although studying illness art or conducting museum tours is

1 Notable exceptions have already been documented in this book from Christine Borland, Stella Bolaki, Jay Baruch and Kelli Auerbach, Laura Ferguson and Katie Grogan, and Rutherford. See the Bibliography for details on these resources.

gaining traction, rarely is *making* part of the learning program. When arts methods are employed in health contexts, they are far more likely to be conducted with patients rather than healthcare learners and professionals.[2] I hypothesize that there may be structural barriers, a lack of collaboration with artists, or simply not knowing how art could be a valid methodology to study illness that has caused this absence of research-creation. I seek to overcome each of these barriers in my "Book as Body" pedagogical design.

The particular structuring of these workshops is meant to demonstrate how research-creation can be thoroughly included in academic and community health humanities contexts alike, and expand notions of what kinds of artistic inquiry are feasible within a standard classroom set up. Acknowledging the inherent structural, safety, and financial obstacles of conducting fine arts outside of specialized arts studios, I will show how nontoxic workshops can take place in a wide variety of settings and with minimal overhead. I will then investigate specific artists' books that the participants made, and how these works utilize and subvert aspects of bookness to elucidate their own complex lived experiences of symptoms. Finally, I will incorporate the feedback I received from the participants into my analysis of the workshop outcomes.

"Book as Body" Workshop Outline

The following is a detailed outline of my workshop procedure. It is meant to serve as a guide for others who wish to conduct their own research-creation or artist's book workshop. It must be noted that even though I am deeply entrenched in this artistic practice, with over a decade of personal, academic, and pedagogical experience, I still partnered with a medical humanities professor, Dr. Stella Bolaki, to round out the leadership expertise. I believe co-teaching ultimately led to the depth of knowledges necessary to enhance participant buy-in and for the ultimate success of

2 Kimberly Fraser and Fatima al Sayah, "Arts-Based Methods in Health Research," *Arts & Health* 3 (2011): 110–145.

this workshop. I strongly advise this kind of arts and medicine partnership within the foundations of any interdisciplinary health humanities venture.

Goals

The overarching goal of this workshop is to investigate how artists' books can foster productive communication and relationality between makers and readers. Under this umbrella, I aim to show how a phenomenological engagement of symptoms enables one to more fully express a lived experience as an artist's book than may have been possible through linguistic means alone. My next goal is to demonstrate the potentiality of translating a symptom into a book as a form of research-creation that critically engages with wider societal and institutional implications of health and illness. My final goal is to use these artists' books as a catalyst to formulate embodied knowledge—spoken, visual, performative, and tactile—for generative reflections on particular and collective meanings of illness.

Methodology

The primary methodology for these workshops is phenomenology applied to the making and reading of artist's books. Phenomenology, or the philosophical practice of examining lived experience, is apt for this workshop because it legitimizes the authority to make meaning through one's memories and sensing body. A contemporary feminist phenomenological lens also overtly addresses how geography, racial background, gender, orientation, and socioeconomic status all impact perception.[3] Although we can attempt to perceive a phenomenon or symptom prelinguistically and without interpretation—as pure feeling—these perceptions will always be framed through the particular background and

3 Havi Carel, *The Phenomenology of Illness* (Oxford: Oxford University Press, 2016), 4.

identity of the subject. Acknowledging such subjectivities opens the possibility for one's symptoms to be interpreted in a multiplicity of meanings with and by others. Therefore, the power to interpret illness is flipped from specialized medical knowledge to each maker's own lived experiences. This inversion of authority enables one to recognize the legitimacy of meanings and significances of illness that may be quite different from another's perspective.

Context

I conducted three "Book as Body" artist's book workshops for this study. The first two workshops took place at the University of Kent in Canterbury, England in the Spring of 2019. Of these, one was conducted with the members of the University of Kent Medical Humanities Reading Group, which consists of medical professionals, humanities professors, and health humanities students. The other workshop in Canterbury also took place on the university campus, but was open to community members and academics from any discipline. The workshop structure and content were formed in collaboration with Dr. Stella Bolaki, Professor of English and head of the Medical Humanities Program at the University of Kent.

The theme of the workshop was clearly stated in the marketing materials I used, which included digital fliers and an explanatory text emailed to relevant health humanities groups and listservs, as well as pointed invitations to local health organizations. Dr. Bolaki reached out to the local Pilgrims Hospices, with whom she has an established relationship. It is important that participants understand the potentially sensitive themes of the workshop prior to attendance, so they have the opportunity to respond with any questions or concerns.

The respondents to the open workshop consisted of healthcare professionals, retired healthcare professionals, medical humanities and arts students, humanities academics, and those who identify as living with a chronic illness or have had an acute but profound illness experience. These categories often overlapped. The first workshop with the University of

Kent Medical Humanities Reading Group consisted of five participants, and the open workshop had twelve people in attendance.

The third workshop took place at the CHCI Health and Medical Humanities Network Summer School hosted at the Columbia University Global Centers in Paris, France in the Summer of 2019. This annual summer school is part of a larger medical and health humanities conference. The participants of this workshop consisted entirely of graduate students whose research intersects with the health and medical humanities, regardless of their particular discipline. My workshop was a required component for the summer school, and there were eighteen participants.

Workshop Structure

A strength of the workshop format is its accessibility. My goal is to demonstrate that anyone can create an artist's book that has aesthetic merit and can effectively communicate lived experience. To accomplish this, I first provide a vast range of artistic materials to craft their books because restricting art methods to only drawing or painting can be a barrier for those with anxiety about their "artistic skills." As well, the supplies are relatively inexpensive, highly mobile, low mess, water soluble, and easily stored at home. The artist's books we create don't require specialized equipment, onerous safety considerations, or ventilation systems. Further, the compact size of artists' books ensures the materials can fit into a backpack or carry-on suitcase if the participants have traveled to attend the workshop.

The room set up and supplies were consistent across all three workshops. Before the workshops began, I spread the copious amounts of bookmaking and artistic supplies across the tables. I arranged the room to consist of one long table or tables connected in a "U" formation. In my experience, I find students rarely stand up to explore the room's supplies and tend to only use the materials that are directly in front of them. Therefore, this unifying room layout ensures that everyone can see the wide variety of materials to work with. They can also easily observe each others' variety of creative solutions and receive ongoing feedback from their neighbors to inform and enhance their own ideas.

The first workshop took place in three hours, the second in four hours, and the third workshop spanned five hours. Everyone works at their own pace, and there are comments in each group requesting more or less time. Overall, I recommend four and a half hours for this workshop. Based on other artist's book workshops I have conducted, this ideal length of time would also be split over two days to give the participants a break, the opportunity to bring in additional materials from home, and time for reflection before completing and critiquing their books.

Once everyone arrives, I warm up our discussions with introductions that include a "head-space" statement, that is, what emotions they are experiencing in this moment, what expectations for the day may be, and if there are any outside preoccupations that might prevent them from being totally present. These statements initiate our time together as a space for sharing and listening.

I begin each workshop with a lecture and slide show on the links between books and bodies. I make this link literal with examples of books bound in human flesh, such as Tagny Duff's artist's books and *Burke's Skin Pocket Book* detailed in Chapter 3 of this book. I then summarize the historical intersections between medicine and bookmaking, making note of the collaborative teams that crafted exemplary anatomical tomes.[4] This lecture pays special attention to anatomical flap books, such as physician Johann Remmelin and artist Stephan Michelspracher's *Catoptrum Microcosmicum* (1619), because they exemplify medical learning through multi-sensory books.

Viewing these paper layers of the body, I initiate a "noticing game" to warm up their observational acuity. I ask the participants to describe exactly what they see on the page, which has been projected onto the front of the room. With the bizarre floating organs, volcanic landscape, *memento mori,* and animals surrounding the androgynous nude figure, there is much to describe. I then ask, given the list of denotations we just compiled, what deeper meanings and allegories can be ascribed to this printed body. These connotations may include allusions to biblical figures, gender roles, and mortality. This exercise flexes the participants' description skills

4 Examples of this historical perspective are provided in Chapter 2.

and foreshadows the critique procedure we will employ at the end of the workshop.

Next, I show how contemporary artists express themes of illness, disability, injury, mourning, and doctor–patient encounters through their artists' books, like in Joan Lyon's *The Gynecologist*. I then showcase artist Martha Hall and play a portion of her documentary, "I Make Books."[5] Hall's practice demonstrates how artists' books can initiate and mediate productive communication between patients and physicians. This example makes explicit links to artists' books' potential for a deeper understanding of another's lived experiences by medical professionals and ultimately, more holistic patient care.[6] Finally, I end the lecture by sharing my own artistic collaboration with my sister, Devan Stahl, and the books that we create together.[7] I am able to bring these books into the workshop so the participants may touch, read, smell, and experience artists' books first hand.

Creation Procedure

Although I do not explicitly frame it as such to the participants, I structure the making process as a phenomenological practice based upon the work Maurice Merleau-Ponty[8] and Don Idhe.[9] As outlined in Idhe's book, *Experimental Phenomenology* (1977), the phenomenological procedure can be summarized as feeling, description, imaginative abstraction, and re-interpretation. The first step begins with identifying and inhabiting a sensation or "symptom" felt within the participants' bodies that "precedes classification and systematization."[10] This symptom could be fairly

5 Martha Hall, "I Make Books," interview by Jennifer Tuttle, The Maine Women Writers Collection, University of New England, 2004, film, 18:24, <https://www.youtube.com/watch?v=zQCjsutVAtk>

6 A full account of Martha Hall's books is available in Chapter 5.

7 A full account of this collaboration is provided in Chapter 4.

8 Maurice Merleau-Ponty, "What Is Phenomenology?" in *The Essential Writings of Merleau-Ponty*, ed. Alden L. Fisher (New York: Harcourt, Brace & World, 1969), 28–35.

9 Don Idhe, *Experimental Phenomenology* (New York: Capricorn Books, 1977), 32.

10 Ibid., 32.

innocuous, like blurry shortsighted vision, or more serious bodily preoccupations like facial burns from ongoing cancer treatments. I also explain that psychological concerns or emotions like mourning, anger, and anxiety are also valid options for this workshop, since they too are felt in and through the body.

I emphasize the importance of choosing a *symptom*, rather than a diagnosis, for several reasons. First, it retains a sense of privacy for the makers to discuss a sensation rather than diagnostic label. I want to avoid any preconceived notions or judgments of what a diagnosis entails. A particular symptom, because it can often derive from numerous different ailments, retains a benefit of the doubt to its origins. Second, it allows us to focus on a particular aspect of one's subjective phenomena instead of attempting to encapsulate the myriad symptoms pertaining to a diagnosis. In a four-hour workshop, attempting to portray the global change to one's life during an illness may not be feasible. Finally, the experience of a general symptom is more likely to be shared among the group of participants rather than a specific diagnosis. This is the difference between creating a book on aching knee joints rather than, say, rheumatoid arthritis. Although there are vast volumes dedicated to categorizing and naming our ailments, we are far more likely to be familiar with and even share their relatively narrow set of felt manifestations. In a focus on symptoms, the participants may feel more connected to each other's representations of bodily sensations, consequently increasing the potential for relationality.

Once a symptom has been chosen, the next step in the workshop is to write a private sensory description of the phenomena in as much detail as possible. To aid in this auto-ethnographic pursuit, I developed a list of sensory questions to ask the participants. Although the questions may seem peculiar and inapplicable at first glance, I encourage them to come up with an answer for each one. The questions ask participants to open their imaginations and give new language to a familiar sensation. Since we won't be sharing these lists, I encourage their answers to be as personal, strange, and honest as possible.

- Let's start with how your symptom feels. What is the texture of your symptom? Sandpaper, rough, sharp, prickly, smooth, slippery, or velvet? What is its pressure? Swollen, tight, hard, constricting, stiff, or loose, give under pressure, wobbly, unsteady? What temperature is it? Burning, soothing warm, cold like metal, or icy? What is its weight? Is it heavy, dragging you down, can you carry it in your arms without effort, or does it float above you? How pervasive is its feeling? Is it full of sensation or numbing? Is it always lurking in the background, periodically bursting forth, or constantly known?

- What does it sound like? Loud, crunchy, hollow, thudding, knocking, crackling, or booming; or does it absorb sound, damped it, or is it silent? Does it make a sound that others can hear, or just inside your own body or mind?
- How do you see your symptom? Is it blurry, obscured, hidden, an empty space where something should be; or obvious and you can't hide away? What size is it? Do you look at it through a microscope or can you hold it in your hand, carry it in a backpack, does it surround your entire body, or is it as big as a building? Does it actually fluctuate in size? What color is it? Is it solid color from a crayon box, sliding from one color into another; or iridescent, shimmery, or glittery?
- What does it taste like? Metal, sour, foul, spicy, bile, spicy heat, citrus sour, sweet like a candy, like menthol, or nothing at all?
- What does it smell like? Citrus, mint, woody pine, cooking spices, floral, sweet like a bakery; or rotting, chemicals, ammonia, astringent alcohol, smoke, or bodily smells?
- How does your symptom move? Does it beat to a rhythm or vibrate? Is its movement unpredictable, chaotic, or regimented? Does it sway, curl, bounce, or swirl? Does it slip through your body like falling sand? Where does your symptom reside? If inside your body, where? Does it travel around, stay still, or grow into other parts?

Once the introspective descriptions are compiled, the next step in the phenomenological practice is to move outside of the body to describe the ways the symptom moves outwards: impacts to daily life, relationships with others, and future plans. It also encompasses what may be a fairly benign symptom in the present, but nevertheless imposes an immense psychological weight of imagining how it may progress. These questions begin to move beyond immediate description and into ascribing meaning to a particular sensation.

- Does your body move through space differently now because of this symptom? How? Are there spaces you no longer have access to? Are there new spaces you frequent?
- Are there tools you can no longer use or substitutions you have made to accomplish tasks? Have you invented new tools and techniques?
- Has your symptom stopped you from doing certain things you used to enjoy? Have you taken up new activities?
- How have your future plans changed because of this symptom?
- How has this symptom impacted your relationships with family, friends, and people you just meet? Is this symptom something you generally keep secret from others? Have some relationships fallen away, and have others strengthened?

It is important that this line of questioning does not simply frame illness and the experience of symptoms as a series of losses, but also brings to light the creativity and affirming aspects of living through hardships.

Equipped with this extensive list of descriptors, the participants can begin to imagine how a symptom can take the form of a book. For example, many of the words they use to describe their bodies can be likewise communicated through material and touch. If a participant described her dry eyes' texture as "rough," she may choose to make her book out of sandpaper to wordlessly express this sensation to the reader. If one focuses on elbow pain, they might reconceive the spine of the book into the hinged movement of an arm. These creative translations may not have been possible without first detailing all the ways a phenomenon is felt and known through the senses.

Since the translation of their chosen symptom into an artist's book may still be ambiguous at this point, I share my own bodily artist's book,

Crunchy Knees, as a concrete example of this practice (see Figure 1.1). This book communicates my own felt symptom of crunchy, loud knees. I began making this sculptural book by sectioning off half of the book's pages and folding them into a staircase shape, which expresses where I am most acutely aware of the loud crunch of my knees at every step. These steps are colored as a progression from yellow to red, recalling the progression of my symptom and its potentially painful future.

The other half of my book is wrapped in a wrinkled, flesh-like cloth. Along the median of this section runs a longitudinal, protruding stitch. This scar of bound skin foreshadows the prospect of future knee surgery. Finally, picking up the book by this section, one may be startled to hear its loud crunch. Between the wrapped pages hides a mass of crinkled plastic, which uncannily crunches in a similar resonance with my knees.

The elements of this book culminate in a multi-sensorial experience of what is like to live with the symptom of crunchy knees. In it, I represent the present state of my body and how I see this symptom affecting my body in the future. I point out to the participants that I did not have to write about my knee in order to give the reader of my book a sense of it. I also did not need to draw a picture of a knee, but instead I made use of the book's hinge to signify the movements of this joint. The challenge here is not to *illustrate* the body necessarily, but for the book to *become* a bodily referent. I encourage the participants to think abstractly in this way while reiterating that the workshop is also completely open to any manner of expression that the participant deems accurate and representative of their own particular experience.

A main aspect of the bookmaking workshop is to show the participants how to craft a handmade book. However, books that make use of multiple folios and signatures are also time intensive, difficult to bind in one's first attempt, use large amounts of potentially expensive paper, and can form what may be an overwhelming number of pages to effectively transform into a single symptom. Therefore, I have found that the simple "zine" fold is optimal for the structure of this workshop because it makes extremely efficient use of material and time. The participants need only to fold and cut a single large sheet of multi-media fine art paper in order to form a book with three full spreads and a front and back cover—no binding required.

This fold is simple enough for the participants to repeat at home with any size or kind of paper so they may continue a bookmaking practice in their own time. The majority of the workshop, at least two hours, is spent transforming this initial empty zine book into an external manifestation of their lived experience.

As the participants begin experimenting with the cornucopia of art supplies before them, I reiterate the idea that paper is a skin, and when we fold it, we are creating a dimensional exterior and interior home for the body and thoughts. I ask participants to consider how their symptom would look if a piece of paper were to physically experience it. How can they fold, encase, hide, layer, expand, stuff, glue, expose, tear apart, ball up, color, alter, destroy, build upon, texturize, or emboss this paper to express their symptom? I ask if it is better to transform the book into a static sculpture to show a profound moment, or utilize the turning of a page as a signal for duration.

While making their books, I play classical music and roam the room fielding questions and giving one-on-one feedback on the development of their ideas. I ask each participant if they need technical or conceptual assistance. The music provides a bit of privacy for our discussions and I reiterate that it is not necessary for them to explicitly disclose their symptom in order for me to assist their progress. As an experienced arts instructor, I offer the workshop participants my technical expertise and guidance throughout the creation process.

The final hour of the workshop is reserved for a roundtable critique of their newly formed artists' books. If the group is larger, like the CHCI workshop in Paris, I split the group and ask a co-instructor to lead the critique for half of the participants in another room. I want to make sure each book has about five minutes of collective reflection within the overall timeframe of the workshop.

The participants sit in a circle holding their books, and I ask them to hand their book to the person on the left. I give a minute for them to explore the new book they are holding before commencing the critique. Instead of the participant explaining their own book to the group, the neighbor who is holding the book is given the first opportunity to describe the book, walk us through its contents, and offer an interpretation of what they think the book may mean. The discussion is then open for others to provide their own interpretation or point out details that may have been missed in the first reading. Finally, the floor is given to the artist if they have a response to the discussion occurring around the meaning of their artist's book. However, the artist is under no obligation to offer any further explanation. This structure of critique ensures each artist retains a sense of privacy surrounding the particularities of their book's inspiration while still inviting the group to collectively reflect on its perceived meaning.

If there is time remaining, I find it useful to receive group feedback on how the workshop went: if they enjoyed this activity, if they found it useful to examine their bodies anew, what it was like to listen to others discuss their books, what it meant to transform their bodies into a book, and finally, what was surprising or insightful about the workshop. After this group analysis, I ask them to fill out individual anonymous feedback forms with similar questions but with more emphasis on how this workshop can be improved in the future.

Mobilizing Bookness in Bodily Expression

The book medium proved to be a productive format to communicate lived experiences of symptoms as the participants utilized a full range and diversity of bookness. To accomplish these expressive feats, the participants capitalized on and created tensions between form, material, sensory interaction, text, narrative, temporality, and performativity. These aspects of bookness also contributed to the practice of phenomenology by materializing the inward- and outward-facing effects of symptoms, and then the relationality between subjects as we experienced them together in the group critique. This next section examines their creative solutions to the workshop prompt before moving on to the philosophical implications of this bookmaking practice.

Form

The forms of the books ranged from traditional codices to completely abstracted sculptures with little-to-no reference to the original book shape. Of course, the traditional book forms proved to be more straightforward for the reader to navigate and understand as a progression of time or narrative. The sculptural books, however, often confounded the reader as the typical gesture of turning pages became obstructed or impossible. We often asked, "How do we read a book without pages?"

One such sculptural book engaged the symptom of blurry vision. The artist formed a large, white, cloud-like mass atop red paper in the center spread of her book, which prevented the reader from fully viewing the other page spreads. This mass could also be described as a pin cushion, since numerous colorful sewing pins were stuck into the form. We as readers are given more insight into the meaning of this book by looking at its front and back covers, which are populated with layers of iridescent discs and a floral motif. When describing her book, the artist explains:

> I have some eye problems [...]. After several examinations, [the optometrist] figured out, actually, there are some wastes my eyes, which naturally I was born with and it kind of reflects the light that goes into my eyes [...]. I think those little plastic circles, like the wastes in my eyes, kind of reflect light. And this [sculpture] is the fear of going through a cataract operation. Those [red colors underneath] are blood. This fear also prompts me to study Early Modern description and surgical experience for my dissertation. I probably read too many sixteenth century descriptions of sharp objects going into the eye. So it's very literal to my body. Basically, a cataract is kind of a white jelly in the eye and opaque like this [sculpture].[11]

The artist exemplifies how purposefully obstructing an aspect of bookness, like viewing pages, evokes a reader's awareness to the parallel prospect of blindness. As the concern of impending blindness becomes a preoccupation, or *dys-appears*, as Drew Leder would say,[12] so too is the reader's attention focused on this concern. Although a traditional book

11 Anonymous workshop participant, group critique by Darian Goldin Stahl, Paris, June 17, 2019.

12 Drew Leder, *The Absent Body* (Chicago: The University of Chicago Press, 1990), 88.

uses the turning of pages to progress a narrative, this book's prickly obstruction transfers the fear of not being able to see or read onto the reader, fostering an embodied perception of this feeling. As a single momentous sculptural form, this book merges the artist's research on historical eye operations, present fear of going blind, and future prospects of surgical interventions all at once.

Materiality

Another aspect of bookness the participants used to foster meaning was materiality, that is, how the materials incorporated into the pages and covers formed literal and conceptual links between subjects. Some artists did this by thoughtfully incorporating atypical media into their books as material signifiers for how a symptom feels. For example, one participant formed a multi-layered enveloping of progressively smaller books, whose center is slowly revealed to contain a small pebble. He explained that a small growth sits at the base of his coccyx, "and it always feels like [he is] sitting on a pebble and it's hidden inside many little layers" of his body.[13]

Another artist formed her book out of dark paper with light flecks that looks similar to soil, and incorporated a sculpture of a mushroom to recall the dissolution of self she experiences during a seizure. The first interpreter of this book intuited the reference to fertile soil by stating, "So when I opened up, the first page says, 'If I Die,' and to me, I'm always reading it as a landscape."[14] In response to this interpretation, the artist explains:

> I love the reading with it as a landscape. This is about a seizure, which I've had a few of in my life. […] This thing in the middle, just so everyone's aware, it's based on a mushroom that bleeds. […] This was like the feeling of being drawn into the earth. But I've had this experience. It's like, I've kind of been sucked into my surroundings. I can't distinguish my body from the earth.[15]

13 Anonymous workshop participant, group critique by Darian Goldin Stahl, Canterbury, April 10, 2019.

14 Anonymous workshop participant, Paris, June 17, 2019.

15 Ibid.

The author effectively uses the combination of earth, mushroom, and the short text, "If I Die," to express the feeling of losing her sense of bodily containment. This book also foreshadows a time when she may not recover from an experience of another seizure and becomes a part of the earth. Her use of materials communicates a sense of mortality and joins all of us as readers into the knowledge that our material bodies will one day transform and absorb into other forms of life.

Senses

Although artists' books are inherently multi-sensory, some of the artists in the workshops focused heavily on a sensory reading of their books to construct their meaning. One artist relied on imaginative eye colors to contrast his emotions of both exhaustion and exuberance during Pride Month. The first interpreter of this book detailed its contents:

> Here is the first page, and these are very irritated and watery looking eyes with reflective pupils. So, my reading, I guess, is that whatever is happening in the world has kind of produced this state of inflammation and sadness. [...] And then the final images are these eyes that, while they do seem to resonate with the first one and that there's been sort of bags that are under them, they are very brightly colored—they are rainbow. And they have stars as pupils, which are still reflective but seem to be less about maybe throwing back whatever is coming in, but about taking it in and seeing something divine in them.[16]

Another artist used the contrast of color to speak toward issues of identity, discrimination, and her symptom of frustration. The cover of her book shows white lace glued over black paper. The internal contents show two photographs of classrooms, one vintage and one contemporary, both portraying People of Color grouped and sequestered to the edge of the classroom. The final back cover of the book portrays a zebra pattern, which the artists explains is meant to represent Black and white persons living and learning side by side rather than in segregation. In the artist's words:

16 Ibid.

> We've got white kids in the long table like this one, taking classes. And you can see the tiny two Black kids by the side kept all alone. So I bring them social justice in here. You know, bringing them equality in art. Everybody should be included in whatever is going on in the classroom.[17]

The colors used in both of these books heavily influence our reading. In the beginning of each, color connotes the emotional toll of discrimination. The use of rainbow and zebra patterns by the end of the books are not only used to point toward the authors' identities but also toward a more optimistic future of inclusion and equity.

Touch was another way that the artists imparted meaning for their readers. Several participants pierced their pages with pins and needles, which forced a delicate handling. Most often, the pins were used to indicate the symptom of pain—psychological or physical—felt by the author, and also had the potential to impart a very real pain for the readers if they were not careful. For example, one participant relays that she was forced to retire from her career as a physician due to a spinal surgery that left the right side of her body compromised. She could no longer effectively examine patients, and lost her independence with everyday tasks like carrying heavy grocery bags or driving. She represented this bodily and emotional pain as pins piercing through the word "Doctor" written in her book.[18]

Other books used sound to engage the readers' senses. One participant expressed her recent experience of a fever by sonically portraying the symptom of insomnia. She did this by layering multitudes of thin, crinkled paper that the reader is forced to turn over. The artist states, "So we have multiple layers to go through and they make this rustling sound because I couldn't rest at all. And I wanted to express this by rustling."[19] In all of these examples, the authors are attempting to form an embodied connection with the readers through a multi-sensory "reading" of their books. They are using their books to touch the reader, in a very real sense, in order to elicit an empathetic response.

17 Anonymous workshop participant, Canterbury, April 10, 2019.

18 Ibid.

19 Anonymous workshop participant, Paris, June 17, 2019.

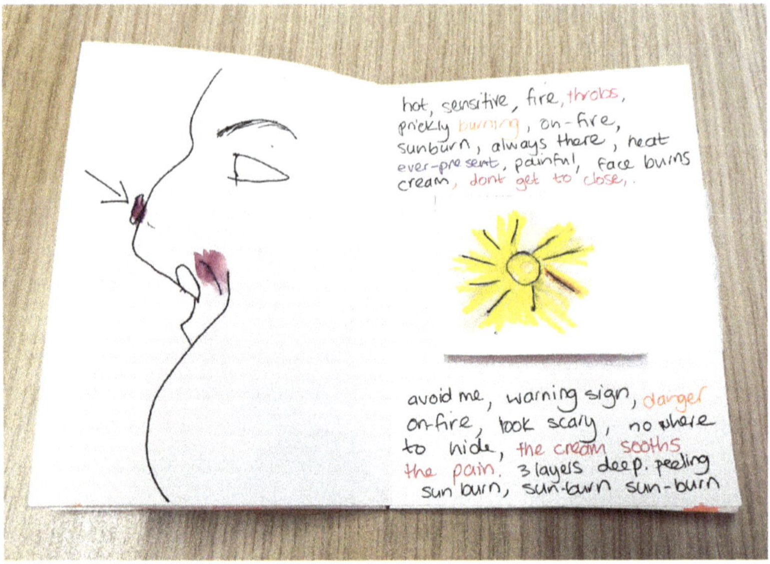

Figure 6.1: Anonymous workshop participant, *Burning Skin*, paper and pen, 6″ × 4″, Canterbury, April 10, 2019.

Text

Although text is not necessarily the focus of this workshop, many participants utilized the tension between words and images. One nurse chose to reformulate her sensory description list to poetically caption her drawings for the symptom of a hot, burning face (see Figure 6.1). Having just undergone skin cancer treatments, this participant drew the red, inflamed skin on her nose and cheeks over and over in her book. Alongside these drawings, she included text like:

> hot, sensitive, fire, throbs, prickly, burning, on-fire, sunburn, always there, heat, ever-present, painful, face burns, cream, don't get to close, avoid me, warning sign, danger, on-fire, look scary, nowhere to hide, the cream soothes the pain, 3 layers deep, peeling, sun burn, sun-burn, sun-burn.[20]

20 Anonymous workshop participant, Canterbury, April 10, 2019.

The incorporation of her sensory text gives the reader a glimpse into both the internal sensations of burning flesh and how the external manifestations of the treatment, an inflamed face, may result in a sense of shame and isolation. The interrelation of personal and interpersonal impacts of these symptoms is made visible through the artist's poetic combination of text and image.

Narrative

Although we tend to think of narrative as text-based, the workshop exemplified how a story can be told in the near-complete absence of words. Through the progressive turning of pages, workshop participants expressed the beginning, middle, and end phases of symptoms. For example, the image-based narrative presented by a participant depicts her loved one's progression through mental distress over the course of its pages. Titled, *What's On My Mind?* the artist collages several cutouts of shirt shapes over the span of her book, which are meant to depict how her loved one changes outfits over and over at the beginning of a manic episode. The initial interpreter tacitly understood that a transformation was occurring over the span of this book: "We're shown three versions of the body in different images. What I appreciate about this is the sense of the body as always changing."[21] The artist then expanded on this initial meaning in our group discussion:

> "What's on my mind?" So for someone who has a mental illness and who's seeking help, that's a question that they feel that everyday everyone's asking them. "So what's going on? What's going through your mind today? How are you feeling today?" Especially anyone who knows the condition can ask them that. So, "What's on *my* mind?" This person is asking back. This [book] is basically what I would think when they are at the peak of mania and so much activity going on. The person shows the mania stages when they keep changing the clothes.[22]

21 Anonymous workshop participant, Paris, June 17, 2019.
22 Ibid.

Although this is a generally wordless artist's book, there is a clear narrative arc. The first outfit shown is bold and surrounded by colorful letters and symbols of lightning bolts to signify hyperactivity. The final shirt is shown against a black background, which the artist explains signals the entrance into the depressive state at the end of her loved one's manic episodes. This exceedingly short narrative nevertheless has much to say: it informs the reader how an inward, psychological symptom goes on to influence one's outward behavior; and finally, how this manifestation of a symptom then signals an outpouring of inter-relational concern and care from others.

Temporality

The participants tacitly understood the inherent temporality of books to propel or stymie a coherent storyline. In one participant's diaristic book, the line, "Take one tablet every day," is repetitively scrawled across the center spread underneath of four actual prescription medications that he pasted onto the page. As the first interpreter explains:

> And then we open it, and we get this date, "July 26, 2016," which obviously must be significant because it's just there on its own. Maybe it's like, reminiscent of a diary entry. Following that we get a recommendation with an asterisk, that this person takes a tablet every day, and "every day" is written repeatedly.[23]

The artist then offered an explanation of a daily ritual:

> It was pretty much about my mental health issues. I've struggled with depression, anxiety, and everything else for a few years now. But I started my therapy on July 26, of 2016. [...] It was a weird experience at first because, having come from an immigrant family, mental health isn't an issue that is talked about. Once I started taking medication, it almost became this weird routine of how medication became this daily performance, routine, that made me really question how useful it really was.[24]

23 Ibid.
24 Ibid.

Even though he didn't quite finish his artist's book, he plans on filling the final blank pages with imagery that "should have to deal with some gay culture, gay issues, but at the same time is very celebratory. [...] Even though you're in this particular moment, you know, you still have some empty pages to fill in, which is a literal materialization of where I've been, but also where I might go."[25] The temporality shown in this artist's book portrays many different kinds of passing time. By referencing a diary, we can interpret that each page is meant to signify a day in his life. However, this pace is significantly disrupted when the repeating words, "every day," fill the space of a single spread. This page effectively portrays the condensing of a much longer period of time, punctuated by the routine of taking yet another dose of his medication. Finally, the blank pages at the end of this book project a future space for his identity and wellbeing to flourish.

Performativity

The final aspect of bookness that the artists use to create bodily connections with their readers is performativity. Rather than a typical turning of pages, some artists constructed their books with more complex methods of navigation that force the reader to slow down and more closely investigate the meaning behind such a structure. For example, one medical student's book appeared quite plain at first: a blank, white paper substrate with a subtle white fringe on its covers. However, once the reader moves into the center spread, she comes across an encased mass of bright red, orange, and yellow tissue paper and the single instruction, "... unfold" (see Figure 6.2). Performing this queue, the reader discovers that the bright papers unfurl into a fiery eruption that can no longer be contained by the book covers. Speaking with its maker, this book is meant to portray his hidden feelings of anxiety in medical school and their potential to explode from within. By performing this book, the reader enacts the burnout that plagues medical students.

25 Ibid.

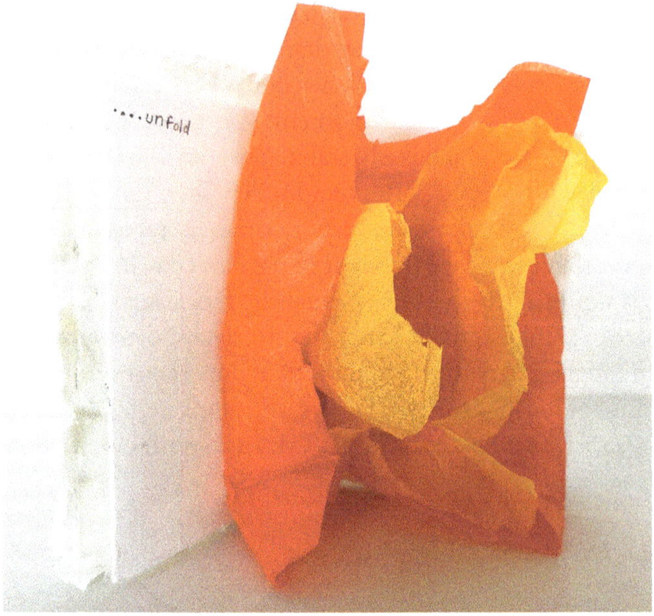

Figure 6.2: Anonymous workshop participant, … *Unfold*, paper, 6″ × 4″, Paris, June 17, 2019.

Another book that must be performed to be understood is a psychiatrist's portrayal of her patients' minds. Recalling the metaphor that the mind is a mysterious "black box," she restructured her book to resemble a black box, with a top flap that the reader must peel back to "read" the contents within. The first interpreter gave this description of the unconventional book:

> It's really fragile. We can feel the vulnerability of it as a body or a mind. So I need to be very careful holding it, and to try to find how to read it and to comprehend it. But if you try to open it like a book you see it is going to collapse. So you need to find another way to read it and look at it. […] I just did try to look from above. I don't know, it's kind of a metacognition thing or psychoanalysis thing, since I know the author.[26]

26 Ibid.

The artist then gave a further explanation for her sculptural book:

> So my first thoughts going into the project were about the "black box" of the mind, and the psyche that I encounter with my patients in psychiatric hospital. So I was thinking in particular about the relationship with the patient, this sort of anxiety being closed up in their mind, and then the difficulties to relate to me, and also to relate to their environment.[27]

As the reader performs this book by pulling back the top and investigating the contents of the "black box," the artist places the reader into her position as a psychiatrist and attempts to read her patients. This confounding book thus effectively portrays both being ill and caring for those who have a mental illness within the same book-body.

Although the prompt for this workshop is to thoroughly investigate a single symptom, what is clear in the description of these books is that they are never solely about one thing. In their reading, the artists show us how one symptom can form a network of personal and interpersonal impacts on one's life. For instance, a book may appear to address the repetitiveness of taking a medication every day, but it also concerns the toll on one's mental health when he is unable to openly communicate his sexuality with his family. Further, although I have categorized these books within particular aspects of bookness, each one could be seen to purposefully subvert more than one element of a traditional book in order to propel its meaning, focus the readers' attention, and form a bodily connection.

Participant Feedback

There were several opportunities to receive feedback about the workshop from the participants. First, through the one-on-one consultations with each participant during the creation of their books. Next, at the end of the workshops when we held a group discussion on the qualities of the

27 Ibid.

workshop. After this, I gave the participants anonymous feedback forms that use a mix of qualitative and quantitative feedback.

Overall, the participants rated their experiences high on a scale from 0 to 5. For instance, the participants rated the background lecture an average of 4.8/5 for exemplifying the creative and communicative potential of artists' books. When asked to rate if this workshop helped them to develop their creative thinking and communication skills, the average score is a 4.5/5. The lowest score was for the question, "This workshop will help me communicate more fully with a clinician as a patient," which received an average score of 3.5. One potential reason for this lowest evaluation could be that the participants would not anticipate taking their books into clinical appointments like Martha Hall. On the other hand, it took several years of a sustained bookmaking practice for Hall to feel confident enough to show anyone other than her immediate family her artist's books. Perhaps with more integration of research-creation in the health humanities, these participants could also feel more comfortable speaking with and through their creations.

Aside from the numerical feedback, I also received written responses to qualitative questions. Some highlights from the "strengths of this workshop" section include:

- Opportunity to explore without expectation.
- Exploring the meaning of words, symptoms from a personal point of view v. doctor's point of view (pain v. sore; raw and blistered v. redness).
- Really appreciated the talks before the workshop to help me understand better the links between books and body in the history of art. I like that it is getting us out of our comfort zone. I like that it doesn't apprehend art in an expressive, not necessarily healing way.
- No binding guidelines, freedom with the form of book.
- The teaching was an eye-opener to my ability to create my piece of work. Articulating and putting down ideas were conveyed to me in the process.

The questions concerning the weaknesses of the workshop almost exclusively involved its length of time, which some deemed too long and others too short. Finally, in the "additional comments" section, participants wrote:

- I loved the teaching process and organization. It helped me start thinking about how powerful colors can be in passing a message.
- I loved this workshop, a powerful and emotive workshop that allowed insightful experiences to be explored in a supportive environment.

While evaluation forms are helpful in some respects, I find the most productive feedback occurs when participants are in the midst of the creative process or communicating the significance of artists' books during the final critique. These recordings and transcriptions are valuable not only to gauge the buy-in and effectiveness of the methods I employ but also to contain the main source of analytical evidence to assess if the goals of the workshop are met.

Philosophical Analysis of the Workshop Outcomes

The workshop's essential provocation, that handmade books express the makers' embodiment, is a research-creation prompt that challenges makers to abstract and materialize the sensations of the body. The "Book as Body" workshops seek to, once again, demonstrate how the practice of phenomenology enables one to elucidate lived experience, and then to use these artists' books as a catalyst to form generative reflections on particular and collective meanings of symptoms. The overarching aim of this research (and this book more generally) is to investigate if and how artists' books foster relationality between makers and readers.

The first steps in a phenomenological practice are to perceive a sensation anew and describe it thoroughly before any kind of cognitive interpretation.[28] It was clear in the group discussion that the sensory description

28 Merleau-Ponty, "What Is Phenomenology?" 28.

prompts from the beginning of the workshop enabled the participants to reconsider a sensation from a novel multi-sensory perspective. One participant noted, "I thought the prompts were really good. You know, what I was working on was something I thought about a lot from a sensory perspective. And still, it's giving me new things to work with that I wouldn't have thought of otherwise."[29]

After description, the next step in the phenomenological practice is to formulate a personal meaning for the perceived sensations. For this particular phenomenological practice, the material intervention of creating an artist's book compels the maker to imaginatively abstract the symptom outside of the body and then re-engage with it through the sensing body so that one may comprehend a lived experience in a new and embodied way. The intertextual translations from sensation to language to book are where the heavy conceptual work of this practice takes place. The step-by-step process of the workshop helped participants make connections between a sensation and aspects of bookness. One participant noted, "It was great, because I think the book is really kind of the bridge between the feeling and the knowledge."[30] Although I take measures for the participants to feel confident in their ability to translate their symptoms into artists' books, I also do not want participants to feel entirely sure how the artists' books would turn out. Leaving room for spontaneity enables the makers to learn *through* the process of making.

As Idhe points out, there is an "essential obscurity"[31] that must occur while one shifts between expressive modalities. Obscurity can open the imagination toward a sense of wonder, experimentation, and embodied learning when we circumvent conventional modes of expression. The abstraction and translation inherent in the workshop's prompt challenges the participants to form original creative solutions through (auto-)ethnographic, sensory, and material research. It is the abstraction that enables both the maker and reader to perceive even habituated sensations as something novel. The generation of new ideas by abstracting the familiar

29 Anonymous workshop participant, Paris, June 17, 2019.
30 Ibid.
31 Idhe, *Experimental Phenomenology*, 18.

through alternative modalities is at this heart of both phenomenological and research-creation practices.

The process of translating a symptom into an artist's book often occurred through an intuitive exploration of the materials rather than conscious linguistic articulations. Taking into account that this group generally had no prior experience in fine art, much less in the medium of artists' books, the sheer variety of materials provided promoted experimentation. As one participant recounts, "I wasn't sure how it was going to come out. But just looking at the materials actually gives you the idea."[32] Another participant adds, "I think for me, it was also generative. And to your point about the materials inspiring the thing, I found a new material that made me think of what the next step was."[33] For both of these makers, the *materials themselves* generated the links between ideas. Released from the confines of channeling all research through language, this embodied way of approaching research furthers the notion that tacit knowledge can reveal itself in the midst of the artistic practices. Creating a book thus invited the makers to explore their own bodies through the materiality of bookness, and how those elements coalesce to convey the meaning of symptoms.

The phenomenological research-creation structure of the workshop not only enabled participants to think about their bodies in new and creative ways during the process of creation, but also enabled a productive collective reflection on the impact of symptoms during the critique. There is a certain amount of trust and vulnerability in letting go of one's creation and opening it for collective critique. I found the obscurity of the artist's book medium to be a benefit in this regard. Without preconceived notions of what a "good" or "bad" artist's book looks like, the participants are less likely to hold their final book to a standard which they may or may not meet. For mixed groups of participants that range from healthcare professionals to students, to laypersons, breaking down hierarchies of knowledge is crucial for open peer-to-peer communication that fosters the feeling that "we are in this together." Because no one was an expert in this medium, I observed more willingness to share the final artist's book with less fear of judgment.

32 Anonymous workshop participant, Paris, June 17, 2019.
33 Ibid.

During the critique, the readers offered multiple and layered interpretations of each other's artists' books due to their abstracted nature. The interpreters formulated meaning through the books' form, content, and perhaps some limited knowledge of the author, while keeping in mind that all of these interpretations were framed through their own life experiences. This step is meant to initiate relational connections between makers and readers by physically handing the book to another person, and focusing our collective attention on its potential meanings. With these many interpretations in hand, we were able to comprehend the wider implications of particular symptoms, and even relate them to our own experiences. What's more, the interpretations offered the artist the opportunity to reconsider their own experiences from new perspectives.

What first became evident in the critique was the significance of receiving these precious handmade objects from their creator. One participant remarked:

> The first thought that came to my mind when I got this is like I'm being given a gift, something I have to unwrap. I sort of have to open it. So that was a feeling of curiosity, also sort of attention that, you know, that it is was given to me.[34]

Another participant notes:

> The thing that struck me first is just how small it is. And because of that there's a kind of intimacy in here. I feel like I'm being led into somebody's inner world. And we really are in such a simple and beautiful way.[35]

The gesture of handing one's book to their neighbor formed an instant relation between maker and reader. These connections then deepened by taking the time and care to consider the book as a materialization of experience.

As conceptualized by Merleau-Ponty, the reversibility of perception encompasses not only how I perceive and how others perceive me, but also how I perceive others perceiving me. This concept was fully witnessed during the artist's book critique, where the author is given the opportunity

34 Ibid.
35 Ibid.

to receive feedback on the significance of their creation to others. One participant noted, "I enjoyed the experience of creating a narrative or reading a symptom, commenting on someone else's symptom, and watching the comments on mine. It kind of made me rethink my interpretation of the symptom I was talking about."[36] The exchange of ideas facilitated by the artist's book clearly formed a reciprocity of attention and care that felt personal and insightful.

After such a focused investigation of their own bodies, it was surprising for many participants to hear how their artists' books stimulated entirely different meanings from others. For example, the "black box" artist's book noted above inspired many possibilities to its meaning. The initial interpreter of this book saw it not as a book at all, but rather "when [he] was looking at it globally, it seemed to [him] like maybe a kind of a ship or something."[37] This interpretation provided an opportunity for the artist to consider how another's perception of a ship could be equally true to her own intention of portraying a black box, and how these interpretations can coexist. The artist responded,

> Is this a black box that I'm trying to open in the therapy, through the development of a relationship to the patient so far, too? There's also a moment of a journey, I thought, a journey and you named it like a ship. And I also kind of like that idea, because in a certain way, you engage on a trip, the missions, and we walk along with the person and sort of do this together.[38]

A phenomenological practice upholds the perception of both the maker and reader to be valid, meaning that, as Idhe states, "all phenomena must be considered 'equally real' within the limits of their givenness."[39] The blending of interpretations for this abstract book demonstrates how widening the possibilities of meaning to include not only the maker's intention but also the subjectivity of each person who reads it, forms an entanglement of relationality that grows to encompass all those who take the time to engage with these artists' books. Because of the layering of meaning

36 Ibid.

37 Ibid.

38 Ibid.

39 Idhe, *Experimental Phenomenology*, 37.

evidenced in the group critique and reflexive dialogue these artists' books sparked on the particular and shared experiences of symptoms, I find the "Book as Body" workshops to successfully meet the preliminary goals.

Pitfalls

My analysis of the artist's book workshops includes some drawbacks as well. First, the workshops only included a total of thirty-five participants. Although this intimate setting allows me to conduct one-on-one feedback with each participant, the overall impact of these workshops on the field of health humanities is, at the moment, also small. The ideal future for these workshops would be to form a replicable model for other collaborative teams of instructors to take up and conduct within their own institutions, positioned within their own expertise and media choices, and thus proliferate generative health humanities research-creation.

The biggest pitfall to demonstrating the transformative, intrinsic value of research-creation is that the participants are self-selected, and therefore already have at least a cursory interest in health humanities. As noted by one physician-participant, the workshop helped her to reconsider the impact of symptoms on her patients' lives, but that other healthcare workers would not generally have the time, or perhaps the will, to conduct such reflexive considerations on their own. She stated,

> [The workshop] really helps you identify and define the aspects of yourself that have been affected, which is not just conventional things. More so it's like exploring taste, smell, the sound, the sensory, and how each condition has that. But we [as physicians] don't consider it because we don't have the time.[40]

Another participant expressed similar sentiments in the anonymous feedback form: "I am not sure the doctor's cabinet would allow for such non-conventional expansion, but if the doctor's cabinet would allow for such non-conventional communication in some shape or form, I think it could be valuable."[41]

40 Anonymous workshop participant, Canterbury, March 25, 2019.
41 Ibid.

To overcome the hurdles of time, and even permission, to engage in phenomenological investigations within the health humanities, Maria Vaccarella argues that "if we want to really strengthen the collaboration with medicine, it has to be really well integrated so it's not just something like 'a little hobby.' "[42] For the most thorough assessment of impact for this kind of workshop, an ideal setting would be as part of a sustained, integrated, and mandatory health humanities curriculum or ongoing education program, where the biases for self-selection are accounted for and everyone has permission to spend their valuable time in creative, reflexive pursuits.

The final pitfall I have identified in the analysis of this workshop concerns an artist's access to perform such health humanities inquiry as a non-medical professional. I have found that it is essential to identify a health humanities scholar or medical professional who *already* champions the value of arts-based inquiry and is willing to put in additional time and effort to integrate art into their outreach and curricula. In this regard, I am grateful for my collaboration with Stella Bolaki and the immense amount of time, professional networks, and experience she brought to these workshops.

Conclusion

Although it is difficult to know the long-term impact of a creative inquiry such as this, it was clear through the qualitative feedback and critique that the participants found value in translating their bodies into books. The combination of the introductory lecture, the use of real-world examples, guided art making, and final critique from an artist invested in the subject matter provided the necessary conditions for the high percentage of buy-in and engagement. Further, aligning the process of this workshop with a phenomenological research-creation practice enabled each person to deeply perceive a bodily sensation. Participants were then able to identify a single symptom's links within a network of personal and interpersonal impacts on their current lived experiences and future plans. Finally, these

42 Maria Vaccarella, interview by Darian Goldin Stahl, Bristol, February 12, 2019.

books acted as a catalyst for understanding the multiple and shared perceptions of health and illness in a collective setting. Because every artist's book is a layering of intention and interpretation, its capacity to simultaneously inhabit multiple meanings between its covers makes this medium an unparalleled generative format.[43] For these reasons, the "Book as Body" workshop has met the overarching goal of exemplifying how artists' books can foster productive communication and relationality between makers and readers.

43 This portion of text was first published: Darian Goldin Stahl, "Field Notes: How To Be Generative," *Synapsis: A Health Humanities Journal* (2019).

Conclusions and Future

Embodied Books exemplifies the many ways artists' books give form and meaning to bodily phenomena. First, creating an artist's book about one's experience of illness is a method of closely investigating one's own body. Such research-creation involves giving renewed attention to sensations that have become habituated, or feelings that are obstinately difficult to fully comprehend, in order to imaginatively give form to the formless. For the participants in the "Book as Body" workshops and artists like Amanda Couch and her artist's book, *Entrail Troyen* (see Figure 4.12), transforming ephemeral sensations into a tangible object had the effect of familiarizing oneself with the mysterious internal. Once externalized, the ways these phenomena impact not only their own bodies, but how they move through the world and plan for the future become more apparent. Thus, creating the book becomes a research-creation methodology of situating a symptom within the much wider network of impacts to one's life, which ultimately gives meaning to what may otherwise feel like random biological occurrences.

For artists and potential makers, I aim for this book to demonstrate the power of translating bodily experiences through artists' books using whatever modalities feel the most accurate. In addition to the vast array of artistic media choices, artists' books also intersect with many other modalities of meaning-making: sensory, textual, image-based, time-based, performative, and material. The sheer versatility of creative choices enables more multi-sensory engagement than almost any other form of art. Also, the accessible nature of folding paper and stacking folios means that most anyone, especially in collaboration with a trusted partner, can create their own artist's book and populate its pages in any manner of communication strategies. When the topics of these books concern the experiences with illness and disability, accessibility is a central consideration. The flexibility of the medium enables each maker to create a book that best expresses their own particular experiences, using the media that best suits their ability and comfort.

Apart from a solely personal meaning-making investigation, artists' books are also a method for makers to reach out and relate to others about their experiences with illness, disability, and encounters with medicine. The mobile life of books ensures the story within reaches far beyond the maker's body and communicates in the absence of her voice. This innate interconnectivity is especially important for circumstances where direct communication is an insurmountable hurdle because the topic is too sensitive or the author is not physically present. For artists like Erin K. Schmidt and her *Unfinished Blanket* (see Figure 4.4), the book serves as an attempt to communicate the incomprehensibility of loss. As the termination of unviable pregnancies remains a taboo topic in our society, as well as death more generally, makers are able to circumvent the need for direct linguistic communication and instead utilize books' sensory modes of meaning-making to express difficult experiences.

For medical personnel, these objects provide an opportunity to engage with honest and uncensored portrayals of illness and how it impacts the lives of patients who may otherwise feel unable to communicate such concerns with their doctors, either because there is no time to do so within the clinical interaction or the concern falls outside of the strictly medical confines of the doctor–patient relationship. Likewise, healthcare workers will not always be able or willing to invest themselves emotionally with each and every patient they meet in person. Making time to engage with patient-made artists' books, physicians and students are able to hold the stories of others from a distanced position, when there are no high stakes for "solving the problem" or "curing the patient." They can simply listen, learn, and be with the patient's story.

Research-creation is further exemplified in this book as a methodology to focus distinct disciplines around their interconnectedness. A parallaxic practice of interdisciplinary collaborators demonstrates how aesthetics form a nexus between scientific, medical, and artistic research. At the intersection of all these disciplines, images are used to evidence bodily phenomena. The layering of this imagery, including medical scans, printed matter, and microscopy, into an artist's book like *Field Notes* exemplifies how research-creation elucidates the interdisciplinary entanglements of health and illness. Therefore, this medium can be employed as vital learning resources across these fields as the images speak to and inform one another.

Mobilizing artists' books as primary pedagogical material exemplifies the intrinsic value of research-creation within medical paradigms. Bookmakers challenge the barriers between medical professionals, stakeholders, and the general public by democratizing what health research looks like. Once bound, the artist's book structure offers a sense of publishable authority to the story within due to books' iconic status in our culture for encapsulating truths and knowledge. The elevated status of the maker's voice as a book is vital for communicating lived experiences not only to those charged in their care but also to broad public audiences who are not privy to specialized medical knowledge or academic journals. Such "resistive potential of art is now being harnessed by social researchers increasingly committed to dismantling stereotypes, accessing the voices of marginalized groups, and engaging in research that propels social change."[1] The accounts of illness presented by artists' books give an authoritative glimpse into the other side of a diagnosis that falls outside of strict clinical boundaries: the impacts to daily life, independence, relationships with others, career opportunities, socioeconomic status, or future prospects; in short, how illness also impacts intersubjectivity and one's way of being in the world.

For the bookmakers profiled, the process of making, including all of the artistic choices, framing, and subject matter, enabled them to gain a sense of authority and control over the meaning of their experiences. Given the vast power differentials between doctors and patients within the clinical setting, where one may be requested to recite a narrative of their private ailments in a harsh sensory environment for near-strangers, all while barely clothed in a hospital gown, it is essential to provide an opportunity for patients to reclaim a sense of authorship to their lived experiences and bodily phenomena at their own pace and in a comfortable space. For those who choose to share their works directly with healthcare workers, like Martha Hall, these artists' books are then found to be capable of sensitizing

1 Patricia Leavy, *Method Meets Art: Arts-Based Research Practice* (New York City: Guilford Press, 2015), 291.

physicians to the needs of their patients. The mediation of abstract books opens the possibility, perhaps counterintuitively, for more direct and honest communication by acting as a stepping-stone between two people. Such feelings of relational understanding are not restricted to a close proximity to or even within the lifetime of their maker, as one's archival book-body will live on and speak volumes as a legacy of lived experience.

Teaching how to create artists' books in health humanities contexts is the final way I demonstrate how research-creation is vital for learning about illness experiences. First, through the hands-on process of translating a sensation into a book form. By practicing a phenomenological process for making books, learners subsequently flex their capacities to understand the subtle ways other artists' books merge text, image, and the senses to communicate. In the health humanities, such pedagogies alert us to how rigid our linguistic-centered communication has become. There are other ways, perhaps even more constructive ways, to communicate one's lived experiences than being prompted to efficiently verbalize the narrative arc of one's illness. Those who hold power in our healthcare systems ought to be well attuned to the myriad methods patients may employ in their attempts to make themselves understood. Bending toward abstract or metaphorical methods of describing bodily phenomena employed by patients, who do not have the benefit of specialized medical knowledge and scientific terminology, will ultimately foster more aligned understandings of illness and goals for living well.

The subjective nature of artists' books promotes a sense of intercorporeality between makers and readers as both parties become implicated in the meaning of these books. Bookmakers evoke an infinite number of relations within a finite object, which sustains their dynamic significance over many different readers. There is the sense that artists' books are in a state of becoming, dependent upon the next interpretation. Although I have made suggestions on how to translate one's body into book form, there is nevertheless no single prescription for making an artist's book nor for determining some kind of "ultimate meaning"—and this is their strength. Just as phenomenology asks us to consider a sensation anew, each artist's book begins a new practice of examination and interpretation. As Merleau-Ponty states, "The unfinished nature of phenomenology and the inchoative atmosphere which has surrounded it are not to be taken as a sign of failure, they were inevitable because phenomenology's task was to reveal the mystery of the world and of reason."[2] Instead of providing concrete answers, artists' books are best utilized to ask more questions: What is surprising about the perspective and experiences portrayed within this book-body? What emotions rise to the surface as you touch this work? What does this artist's book *do* for the production of health knowledge? What is the worth of spending this time? I aim for *Embodied Books* to initiate further dialogues about the worth of research-creation in health humanities contexts as a philosophical and pragmatic method of examining lived illness and disability experiences.

Making and acquiring artists' books is gaining momentum. After dipping in popularity around the 1990s, artists' books are now in the midst of a Renaissance with new programs, collections, and courses established in universities across North America. I assert that the medium's resurgence is not occurring in spite of digital technologies encroaching on the printed page, but because of them. The prediction of digital readers replacing printed text and relegating the book object into obsolescence has sounded for decades, and yet, has not come to pass. The desire to hold a book, smell ink, flip pages, and display a treasured work on one's shelf endures. Our attraction to books is linked to our long cultural history with them to, as Drucker states, "serve as a vehicle to communicate far beyond the limits of an individual life or contacts."[3] When technology advances production into automation and then digitization, a handmade material practice achieves an enticing aura of legacy and artistry. These book objects become all the more precious when they are lovingly crafted by the hands of the author.

However, this is not to say that artists' books are antithetical to technology. Speaking with the artist Veronique Chance about her artist's book, *In the Absence of Running* (see Figure 4.10), she relays that this work is

2 Maurice Merleau-Ponty, "What Is Phenomenology?" in *The Essential Writings of Merleau-Ponty*, ed. Alden L. Fisher (New York: Harcourt, Brace & World, 1969), 43.

3 Johanna Drucker, *The Century of Artists' Books* (New York City: Granary Books, 1995), 8.

presented in exhibitions alongside a tablet that enabled the reader to digitally scroll through "pages" of her arthroscopic knee surgery rather than experiencing them all at once in the massive, unbound-sheet formation of her artist's book. As well, the documentation of my artist's book *Field Notes: How to Be With* also includes a video documentation and recitation so that it can be shared far beyond its five physical editions. On the other hand, the reach and accessibility of digitized versions of artists' books may not hold true in perpetuity. As technology continues to change styles, formats, and hardware, these digital files will inevitably become incompatible or incommodious. For instance, when I visited the Prescriptions Collection at the University of Kent to view Chance's book, the digital tablet version was not included. Chance explained that incorporating a tablet that has to be charged and managed with updates was ultimately incongruous with the archive. The legacy and staying power of this work is in its paper form.

Another way artists' books intersect with digital technologies is through direct download and reassembly. Recalling the practice of unlimited editions of artists' books that could be sent through the mail, initiatives like The Quarantine Public Library give artists the opportunity to upload photocopies of their single sheet zines that visitors to the site can then "freely download, print and assemble—to keep or give away."[4] This repository of books began during the Covid-19 lockdowns as a way to creatively connect people from safe distances. I have taken up this idea in new iterations of my "Book as Body" workshops, and participant-made zines are available to view and download from my own website, <www.embodiedbooks.com>. The flexibility of the artist's book format, even over the internet, fulfills the desire to touch narratives and build community with others over vast distances when physical proximity is an impossibility.

Embodied Books is building toward the integration of research-creation practices in the health humanities. These health contexts may include patient advocacy groups, art therapies, as well as medical classrooms. While

4 Katie Garth and Tracy Honn, "About," Accessed February 21, 2023, <https://www.quarantinepubliclibrary.com/>

creative methods like Narrative Medicine are readily employed in this burgeoning field, arts-based methods are much less often represented. A goal of this monograph is to demonstrate the value of learning with and through creative arts practices, especially for those who hold positions of power to alter curricula and include them in the classroom. I also advocate for collaborative partnerships in these interdisciplinary pursuits to ground the inquiry within a clear and effectual rationale. For a field that is only beginning to include research-creation, we are in the position to shape its future. As we continue to build and configure the health humanities, I argue for making space to conduct the thinking and feeling that can only occur in the midst of making.

From the time artists were dismissed from the anatomical theater in favor of photographic documentation methods, artists' role in medical discourses has generally shifted to critical outsider. Many of the artists profiled here take on this important perspective to reveal the miscommunications, biases, and injustices that continue to pervade Western medical institutions. With the broadening acknowledgment that the greatest medical concerns we face are not entirely biological but also humanistic in how we understand each other in a polarizing world and, primarily, how best to take care, arts and humanities perspectives will continue to become ever more vital within health discourses. From this position *within*, artists and humanities researchers have the potential to transform understandings of illness in partnership with medical practitioners. This shift occurred most notably in the work of Hall, whose artist's books began as a critique of the communication styles of her physicians, and evolved to become primary pedagogical resource material for new generations of medical students.

If we aim to achieve health equity, then the narratives we use to evidence what it is like to move through our healthcare systems must come from diverse perspectives. Those who are empowered with the knowledge and skills to create artists' books then become the arbiters of truth for the stories printed between their covers. The future of this project is to seek out those whose voices are missing from the medical and health humanities collections and curricula and enable them to represent their own authoritative stories in the sharable, archival, and sensitive medium of artists' books. As we grapple with when and how to come together in a post-pandemic society, such artists' books exemplify how research-creation can mediate and generate discourses between health professionals and those who live daily with illness. The multitude of perspectives bound together around a shareable artist's book embodies ways of being-with, even at a distance.

Bibliography

Alexander, Charles. 1995. *Talking the Boundless Book: Art, Language and the Book Arts.* Minneapolis: Minnesota Center for Book Arts.

Barnett, Richard. 2014. *The Sick Rose.* London: Thames and Hudson.

Baruch, Jay M., and Kelli Auerbach. 2012. "Beyond Comfort Zones: An Experiment in Medical and Art Education." *Journal for Learning Through the Arts* 8 (1): 1–14.

Bates, Victoria, Alan Bleakley Bleakley, and Sam Goodman. 2013. *Medicine, Health and the Arts: Approaches to Medical Humanities.* London: Routledge.

Bennett, Jane. 2010. *Vibrant Matter: A Political Ecology of All Things.* Durham: Duke University Press.

Bishop, Jeff. 2008. "Rejecting Medical Humanism: Medical Humanities and the Metaphysics of Medicine." *The Journal of Medical Humanities* 29: 15–25.

Blake, William. 1793. *The Marriage of Heaven and Hell.*

Bleakley, Alan. 2013. "Transitions in Health Humanities: Towards a 'Critical' Health Humanities that Embraces Beauty." In *In/sight 2: Engaging the Health Humanities*, by Lianne McTavish and Pamela Brett MacLean. Edmonton: University of Alberta Department of Art and Design.

Bleakley, Alan. 2015. "When I Say … The Medical Humanities in Medical Education." *Medical Education* 49: 959–960.

Bolaki, Stella. 2016. *Illness as Many Narratives: Arts, Medicine, and Culture.* Edinburgh: Edinburgh University Press.

Bolaki, Stella. 2020a. "Contemporary Artists' Books and the Intimate Asthetics of Illness." *Journal of Medical Humanities* 41: 21–39.

Bolaki, Stella. 2020b. "Artists' Books and Medical Humanities." *Journal of Medical Humanities* 41: 1–5.

Bolaki, Stella, and Egidija Ciricaite. 2017. *Prescriptions: Artists' Books on Wellbeing and Medicine.* London: Natrix Natrix Press.

Carel, Havi. 2016. *The Phenomenology of Illness.* Oxford: Oxford University Press.

Carlin, Jane Anne. 2019. "Artists' Books as Catalysts for Social Change ." *Art Libraries Journal* 44 (1): 2–8.

Carrion, Ulises. 1985. "The New Making of Books." In *Artists' Books: A Critical Anthology and Sourcebook*, by Joan Lyons, 31–44. Rochester: Visual Studies Workshop.

Cartwright, Lisa. 1995. *Screening the Body: Tracing Medicine's Visual Culture.* Minneapolis: University of Minnesota Press.

Chance, Veronique. 2015. *In the Absence of Running.* Canterbury: University of Kent.

Chance, Veronique. 2020. "In the Absence of Running: From Injury and Medical Intervention to Art." *Journal of Medical Humanities* 41 (1): 65–80.

Chapman, Owen, and Kim Sawchuk. 2012. "Research-Creation: Intervention, Analysis and 'Family Resemblances'." *Canadian Journal of Communication* 37 (1): 1–22.

Charon, Rita. 2001. "Narrative Medicine: A Model for Empathy, Reflection Profession, and Trust." *JAMA* 286 (15): 1897–1902.

Charon, Rita. 2008. *Narrative Medicine: Honoring the Stories of Medicine.* Oxford: Oxford University Press.

Ciricaite, Egidija. 2020. "On Photographing Artist's Books." *Journal of Medical Humanities* 41: 81–83.

Classen, Constance. 2012. *The Deepest Sense: A Cultural History of Touch.* Chicago: University of Illinois Press.

Classen, Constance. 2017. *The Museum of the Senses.* London: Bloomsbury Academic.

Cole, Thomas, Nathan Carlin, and Ronald Carson. 2014. *Medical Humanities: An Introduction.* Cambridge: Cambridge University Press.

Connor, Steven. 2004. *The Book of Skin.* London: Reaction Books Ltd.

Costa, Beatriz de, and Kativa Philip. 1989. *Tactical Biopolitics: Art, Activism, and Technoscience.* Cambridge: MIT Press.

Couch, Amanda. 2016. *Entrail Troyan.* Canterbury: University of Kent.

Couch, Amanda. 2020. "Reflections on Digestions and Other Corporealities in Artists' Books." *Journal of Medical Humanities* 41 (1): 7–19.

Crawford, Paul, Brian Brown, Charley Baker, Victoria Tischler, and Brian Abrams. 2015. *Health Humanities.* Hampshire: Palgrave Macmillan.

Davids, Betsy, and Jim Petrillo. 1985. "The Artist as Book Printer: Four Short Courses." In *Artists' Books: A Critical Anthology*, by Joan Lyons, 149–165. Rochester: Visual Studies Workshop Press.

Davis, Duane. 2020. "The Phenomenological Method." In *50 Concepts for a Critical Phenomenology*, by Gail Weiss, Ann L. Murphy, and Gayle Salamon, 3–9. Evanston: Northwestern University Press.

Drucker, Johanna. 1995. *The Century of Artists' Books.* New York: Granary Books.

Drucker, Johanna. 2020. "Bound to Speak: Accounts of Illness in Artists' Books." *Journal of Medical Humanities* 41 (1): 85–88.

Duff, Tagny. n.d. *Cryobook Archives.* Accessed November 4, 2020. <http://tagnyduff.com/projects-current/cryobook-archives/>.

Duff, Tagny. 2011. *Cryobook Archives_Tagny Duff.* February 7. Accessed December 2020. <http://tagnyduff.com/projects-current/cryobook-archives/>.

Duff, Tagny Duff. 2010–Present. *Cryobook Archives.* Montreal.

Ebenstein, Joanna. 2016. *The Anatomical Venus.* London: Thames and Hudson.

Eisner, Elliot W. 1981. "On the Differences between Scientific and Artistic Approaches to Qualitative Research." *Review of Research in Visual Arts Education* 7 (1): 1–7.

Ferguson, Laura, and Katie Grogan. 2017. *Art & Anatomy: Drawings.* New York: University of California Medical Humanities Press.

Finley, Susan. 2008. "Arts-Based Research." In *Handbook of the Arts in Qualitative Research: Perspectives, Methodologies, Examples, and Issues*, by J. Gary Knowles and Ardra L. Cole. Los Angeles: Sage Publications.

Fisher, Linda. 2014. "The Illness Experience: A Feminist Phenomenological Perspective." In *Feminist Phenomenology and Medicine*, by Lisa Folkmarson Käll and Kirstin Zeiler, 33–52. Albany: SUNY Press.

Foucault, Michel. 1976. *The Birth of the Clinic.* Translated by A. M. Sheridan. London: Routledge.

Frank, Arthur. 2018. "Rightness, Place, and Humanistic Health Care Ethics: Fragments of a Moral Inquiry." *GeoHumanities* 4: 310–315.

Fraser, Kimberly Diane, and Fatima al Sayah. 2011. "Arts-Based Methods in Health Research." *Arts & Health* 3 (11): 110–145.

Garland-Thomson, Rosemarie. 2009. *Staring: How We Look.* Oxford, New York: Oxford University Press.

Garth, Katie, and Tracy Honn. 2021. *About.* Accessed February 2023. <https://www.quarantinepubliclibrary.com/>.

Gilman, Sander. 1996. *Seeing the Insane.* Lincoln: University of Nebraska Press.

Grosz, Elizabeth. 1994. *The Volatile Bodies: Toward Corporeal Feminism.* Bloomington: Indiana University Press.

Grosz, Elizabeth. 2004. "Merleau-Ponty, Bergson, and the Question of Ontology." In *Intertwinings*, by Gail Weiss, 13–30. Albany: State University Press of New York.

Guenther, Lisa. 2020. "Critical Phenomenology." In *50 Concepts for a Critical Phenomenology*, by Gail Weiss, Ann L. Murphy, and Gayle Salamon, 11–16. Evanston: Northwestern University Press.

Hall, Martha. n.d. *Prescriptions.* Maine Women Writers Collection, Portland.

Hall, Martha. 1999. *Voices: Five Doctors Speak.* Canterbury: University of Kent.

Hall, Martha. 2000. *The Rest of My Life II.* Maine Women Writers Collection, Portland.

Hall, Martha, Interview by Jennifer S. Tuttle. 2004. "I Make Books." The Maine Women Writers Collection, University of New England. Film, 18:24. <https://www.youtube.com/watch?v=zQCjsutVAtk>.

Hall, Martha, and Martin Antoinette. 2013. *Holding In, Holding On: Artist's Books by Martha A. Hall.* Northampton: Mortimer Rare Book Room, Smith College.

Hansen, Julie, and Suzanne Porter. 1999. *The Physician's Art.* Durham: Duke University Press.

Hasse, Cathrine. 2008. "Postphenomenology: Learning Cultural Perception in Science." *Humanistic Studies* 31: 43–61.

Highmore, N. 1651. *Corporis humani disquisitio.*

Hooker, Claire, and Estelle Noonan. 2011. "Medical Humanities as Expressive of Western Culture." *Medical Humanities* 37 (2): 79–84.

Idhe, Don. 1977. *Experimental Phenomenology.* New York: Capricorn Books.

Idhe, Don. 2008. "Introduction: Postphenomenological Research." *Human Studies* 31: 1–9.

Jennings, M. L. 2009. "Medical Student Burnout: Interdisciplinary Exploration and Analysis." *Journal of Medical Humanities* 30: 253–269.

Käll, Lisa Folkmarson, and Kirstin Zeiler. 2014. "Why Feminist Phenomenology and Medicine?" In *Feminist Phenomenology and Medicine*, by Lisa Folkmarson Käll and Kirstin Zeiler, 8–32. Albany: SUNY Press.

Klima, Stefan. 1998. *Artists Books: A Critical Survey of the Literature.* New York: Granary Books.

Kumagai, Arno K., Elizabeth K. Jones, and Anne L. Kittendorf. 2017. "Creative Art and Medical Student Development: A Qualitative Study." *Medical Education* 51: 174–183.

Lammer, Christina. 2007. "Bodywork: Social Somatic Interventions in the Operating Theaters of Invasive Radiology." In *Visual Interventions: Applied Visual Anthropology*, by Sarah Pink. Oxford: Berghahn.

Leavy, Patricia. 2015. *Method Meets Art: Arts-Based Research Practice.* New York: Guilford Press.

Leder, Drew. 1990. *The Absent Body.* Chicago: The University of Chicago Press.

Leder, Drew. 1992. "Introduction: The Body in Medical Thought and Practice." *Philosophy and Medicine* 43: 1–12.

Leder, Drew. 2016. *The Distressed Body: Rethinking Illness, Imprisonment, and Healing.* Chicago: The University of Chicago Press.

Lepine, Lisa A., Susan D. Hillis, Polly A. Marchbanks, Lisa M. Koonin, Brian Morrow, Burney A. Kieke, and Lynne S. Wilcox. 1998. *Hysterectomy Surveillance—United States. 1980–1993.* MMWR Surveillance Summaries. Semptember 19. Accessed January 2022. <https://www.cdc.gov/mmwr/preview/mmwrhtml/00048898.htm>

Lin, Jenny. 2012. *Skinny Leg.* Montreal.

Lippard, Lucy R. 1973. *Six Years: The Dematerialization of the Art Object from 1966 to 1972.* New York: Praeger Publishers.

Lippard, Lucy R. 1985. "The Artist's Book Goes Public." In *Artists' Books: A Critical Anthology*, by Joan Lyons, 45–48. Rochester: Visual Studies Workshop.

Louie, Patricia, and Rita Wilkes. 2018. "Representation of Race and Skin Tone in Medical Textbook Imagery." *Social Science & Medicine* 202: 38–42.

Loveless, Natalie. 2019. *How to Make Art at the End of the World: A Manifesto for Research-Creation.* Durham: Duke University Press.

Lyons, Joan. 1985. *Artists' Books: A Critical Anthology and Sourcebook.* New York: Visual Studies Workshop Press.

Lyons, Joan. 1989. *The Gynecologist.* Rochester.

Macnaughton, Jane. 2011. "Medical Humanities Challenge to Medicine." *Journal of Evaluation in Medical Practice* 17 (5): 927–932.

Macnaughton, Jane, and Havi Carel. 2016. "Breathing and Breathlessness in Clinic and Culture: Using Critical Medical Humanities to Bridge an Epistemic Gap." In *The Edinburgh Companion to the Medical Humanities*, by Anne Whitehead and Angela Woods, 294–309. Edinburgh: Edinburgh University Press.

Manning, Erin. 2016. "Ten Propositions for Research-Creation." In *Collaboration in Performance Practice*, by Noyale Colin and Stefanie Sachsenmaier. London: Palgrave Macmillan.

Main Women Writers Collection. n.d. *Martha A. Hall Collection 1971–2011.* University of New England. Accessed August 2020. <https://library.une.edu/mwwc/collections/collections-a-z/martha-a-hall-collection-1998-2003/>.

McNiff, Shaun. 2008. "Art-Based Research." In *Handbook of the Arts in Qualitative Research: Perspectives, Methodologies, Examples, and Issues*, by J. Gary Knowles and Ardra L. Cole. Los Angeles: Sage Publications.

Meli, Domenico Bertoloni. 2017. *Visualizing Disease: The Art and History of Pathological Illustration.* Chicago: The University of Chicago Press.

Merleau-Ponty, Maurice. 1968. *The Visible and the Invisible.* Evanston: Northwestern University Press.

Merleau-Ponty, Maurice. 1969. "Eye and Mind." In *The Essential Writings of Merleau-Ponty*, edited by Alden F. Fisher, 252–286. New York: Harcourt, Brace & World.

Miller, Cathleen, and Jennifer Tuttle. 2017. "'I make books so I won't die': Artists' Books in the Archives and in the Classroom." In *Prescriptions: Artists' Books on Wellbeing and Medicine*, by Stella Bolaki and Egidija Ciricaite, 11. London: Natrix Natrix Press.

O'Connell, Helen E., Kalavampara V. Sanjeevan, and John M. Huston. 2005. "Anatomy of the Clitoris." *Journal of Urology* 179: 1189–1195.

O'Connor, Emma. 2015. *S:ST298.402.* Canterbury: University of Kent.

Petherbridge, Deanna, and Ludmilla Jordanova. 1997. *The Quick and the Dead: Artists and Anatomy.* Manchester: Cornerhouse Publications.

Phillips, Michael. 2018. "Printing in the Infernal Method: William Blake's Method of 'Illuminated Printing.'" *Interfaces* 39: 67–89.

Pink, Sarah. 2015. *Doing Sensory Ethnography*. 2nd Edition. Los Angeles: Sage Publishing Ltd.

Prendeville, Jet Marie. 2009. "Livres d'artistes: 1918 to 2000: A Very Special Collection." *The Flyleaf* 56 (1): 4–11.

Radstake, Maud. 2007. *Visions of Illness: An Endography of Real-Time Medical Imaging*. Utrecht: Eburon Delft.

Remmelin, Johann. 1619. *Catoptrum Microcosmicum*. Ausburg.

Rosenbloom, Megan. 2021. *Dark Archives: A Librarian's Investigation into the Science and History of Books Bound in Human Skin*. New York: Picador.

Rouncefield, Mary. 2013. *Mr. Darcy's Advice the Hip Patient*. Canterbury: University of Kent.

Rouncefield, Mary. 2016. "Mr. Darcy's Advice to the Hip Patient." In *Prescriptions: Artists' Books on Wellbeing and Medicine*, by Stella Bolaki and Egidija Ciricaite, 83. London: Natrix Natrix Press.

Rutherford, Emer Ford, Jacqueline Priego-Hernandez, Aurelia Butcher, and Clare Wedderburn. 2018. "Using Photography to Enhance GP Trainees' Reflective Practice and Professional Development." *Journal of Medical Humanities* 44 (3): 158–164.

Sameshima, Pauline, Patricia Maarhuis, and Sean Wiebe. 2019. *Parallaxic Practice: Multimodal Interdisciplinary Pedagogical Research Design*. Wilmington: Vernon Press.

Scarry, Elaine. 1985. *The Body in Pain: The Making and Unmaking of the World*. Oxford: Oxford University Press.

Schmidt, Erin. n.d. *The Unfinished Blanket*. Accessed June 12, 2020. <https://www.erinkschmidt.com/theunfinishedblanket.html>.

Schmidt, Erin. 2016. *The Unfinished Blanket*. Canterbury: University of Kent.

Shapiro, Johanna. 2009. "Medical Humanities and Their Discontents: Definitions, Critiques, and Implications." *Academic Medicine* 84 (2): 192–198.

Sleigh, Charlotte, and Sarah Craske. 2017. "Nine-Tenths of the Iceberg: Research as the Unseen Component of Artists' Work." Interalia Magazine: 1. November. Accessed January 2021. <https://www.interaliamag.org/articles/sarah-craske-charlotte-sleigh-nine-tenths-iceberg-research-unseen-component-artists-work/>.

Springgay, Stephanie, Anise Truman, and Sara MacLean. 2019. "Socially Engaged Art, Experimental Pedagogies, and Anarchiving as Research-Creation." *Qualitative Inquiry* 5 (1): 1–11.

Squier, Susan Merrill. 2007. "Beyond Nescience: The Intersectional Insights of Health Humanities." *Perspectives in Biology and Medicine* 50 (3): 334–347.

Stacey, Jackie. 1997. *Teratologies*. London: Routledge.

Stafford, Barbara Maria. 2007. *Echo Objects: The Cognitive Work of Images.* Chicago: The University of Chicago Press.

Stahl, Darian Goldin. 2014. *The Importance of Dualism.* Wellcome Collection, London.

Stahl, Darian Goldin. 2019a. "Field Notes: How to be Generative." *Synapsis: A Health Humanities Journal.* July 7. Accessed April 7, 2021. <https://medicalhealthhumanities.com/2019/07/07/synapsis-in-paris-field-notes-how-to-be-generative/>.

Stahl, Darian Goldin. 2019b. *Field Notes: How to Be Generative.* July 7. Accessed January 2021. <https://medicalhealthhumanities.com/2019/07/07/synapsis-in-paris-field-notes-how-to-be-generative/>.

Stahl, Darian Goldin. 2020. *Field Notes: How to Be With.* Montreal.

Stahl, Devan. 2018. *Imaging and Imagining Illness: Becoming Whole in a Broken Body.* Eugene: Cascade Books.

Stewart, Elizabeth A., Lynne T. Shuster, and Walter A. Rocca. 2012. "Reassessing Hysterectomy." *Minnesota Medicine* 95 (3): 36–39.

Tarlow, Sarah. 2018. "Curious Afterlives: The Enduring Appeal of the Criminal Corpse." *Mortality* 21 (3): 210–228.

Tarlow, Sarah, and Emma Battell Lowman. 2018. *Harnessing the Power of the Criminal Corpse.* London: Palgrave Macmillan.

Toombs, S. Kay. 1987. "The Meaning of Illness: Phenomenological Approach to the Patient-Physician Relationship." *Journal of Medicine and Philosophy* 12: 219–240.

Toombs, S. Kay. 1988. "Illness and the Paradigm of the Lived Body." *Theoretical Medicine* 9: 201–226.

Toombs, S. Kay. 1990. "The Temporality of Illness." *Theoretical Medicine* 11: 227–241.

Toombs, S. Kay. 1992. "The Body in Multiple Sclerosis: A Patient Perspective." In *The Body in Medical Thought and Practice*, by Drew Leder, Vol. 43, 127–137. London: Kluwer Academic Publishers.

Tuttle, Jennifer S., and Cathleen Miller. 2020. "Unruly Voices: Artists' Books and Humanities Archives in Health Professions Education." *Journal of Medical Humanities* 41: 53–64.

Vaughan, Kathleen. 2005. "Pieced Together: Collage as an Artist's Method for Interdisciplinary Research." *International Journal of Qualitative Methods* 4 (1): 27–52.

Verbeek, Caro, and Cretien van Campen. 2013. "Inhaling Memories: Smell and Taste Memories in Art, Science, and Practice." *Senses and Society* 8 (2): 133–148.

Verbeek, Peter-Paul. 2008. "Obstetric Ultrasound and the Technological Mediation of Morality: A Postphenomenological Analysis." *Human Studies* 31: 11–26.

Vesalius, Andreas. 1540. *De humani corpo ris fabrica epitome.*

Washington, Harriet A. 2006. *Medical Apartheid: The Dark History of Medical Experimentation on Black Americans from Colonial Times to the Present.* New York: Harlem Moon Broadway Books.

Waugh, Patricia. 2018. "Afterward: Evidence and Experiment." In *The Edinburgh Companion to the Critical Medical Humanities,* by Anne Whitehead and Angela Woods. Edinburgh: Edinburgh University.

Weiss, Gail. 2004. *Intertwinings.* Albany: State University Press of New York.

Westminster Medical Society. 1829. "Supplement to Myology." *The Lancet* 11 (no): 468.

Whitehead, Anne, and Angela Woods. 2016. *The Edinburgh Companion to the Medical Humanities.* Edinburgh: Edinburgh University Press.

Wijdicks, Eelco. 2020. "The Galling and Gifted Franz Joseph Gall." *The Lancet: Neurology* 19 (10): 812–813.

Woods, Angela. 2011. "The Limits of Narrative: Provocations for the Medical Humanities." *Medical Humanities* 37 (2): 73–78.

Young, Iris. 1994. "Comments on Seyla Benhabib, Situating the Seld." *New German Critique* 62: 165–172.

Index

Medical Humanities: Criticism and Creativity

Series Editors: Maria Vaccarella, MA, PhD, Senior Lecturer in Medical Humanities, University of Bristol and Kimberly R. Myers, MA, PhD, Professor of Humanities and Medicine, Penn State College of Medicine

This series showcases innovative research, creativity and pedagogy in the interdisciplinary field of medical humanities. Books in the series explore the complexities of human bodies, minds, illness and wellbeing through analytical frameworks derived from humanistic disciplines and clinical practice. The series publishes a range of materials, including monographs and edited collections on scholarly approaches to medical issues in culture; creative works (accompanied by analytical and educational materials) that engage with medical humanities themes; and critical, engaged or radical pedagogies on focused topics for learners in the medical and health humanities.

Medical Humanities: Criticism and Creativity is intended to provide an informative exchange across disciplines, encouraging theoretical and personal reflections on the condition of the human mind/body and contributing to debates on health-related issues from a broad range of perspectives. The series also invites research that opens up critical conversations on being human at the intersection of other forms of humanistic knowledge, such as environmental and digital humanities. We are especially interested in collaborations between academics in the humanities and healthcare professionals.

All book proposals and manuscripts undergo rigorous peer review prior to acceptance and publication.

(Oregon Health and Science University), Barry Saunders (University of North Carolina School of Medicine), Johanna Shapiro (University of California, Irvine, School of Medicine), Marina Tsaplina (The Betes Organization), Craigan Usher (Oregon Health and Science University), Neil Vickers (King's College London), Martin Willis (Cardiff University), Charlotte Wu (Boston University School of Medicine)

Kimberly R. Myers (ed.), *Breast Cancer Inside Out: Bodies, Biographies & Beliefs*.
2021. ISBN 978-1-78874-733-2.

Lisbeth Frølunde, Louise Phillips and Maria Bee Christensen-Strynø, *Moving along: A co-produced graphic novel about Parkinson's dance.*
2023. ISBN 978-1-80079-934-9.

Darian Goldin Stahl, *Embodied Books: Experiencing the Health Humanities through Artists' Books.*
2024. ISBN 978-1-80079-816-8.